Anti-Aging Habits:
137 smart and sassy ways to add years to your life and life to your years

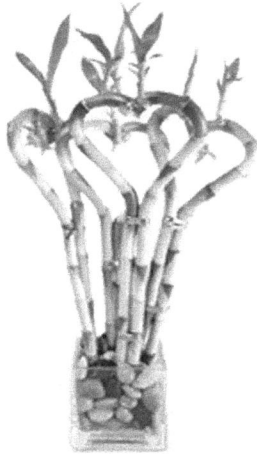

Filomena D. Warihay, Ph.D.

Published in Ft Myers, FL by Stay Young 4Ever, LLC

ISBN 978-0-9641834-9-0

How many 77-year-old women look like this?

The author of Anti-Aging Habits does!

Here, she shares her personal experience showing that you can form new life-extending and life-enhancing habits in just 21 days.

She has spent the past two years conducting research and working with geriatric specialists to validate what she has learned and applied. Her secrets are yours in the pages of the *Anti-Aging Habits* - a powerful, practical you-can- do-it, how-to-do-it guide for anyone who wants to do everything possible to ensure both longevity and good health. Unlike medical tomes or research-oriented reports, *Anti-Aging Habits* is a smart, savvy and sassy guide to happy, healthy, hardy longevity.

It is a first-hand account of how to stay youthful, healthy, vibrant and vital by a 77-year-old woman who **is** youthful, healthy, vibrant and vital.

Anti-Aging Habits will lead readers to a heartier, healthier, happier life.

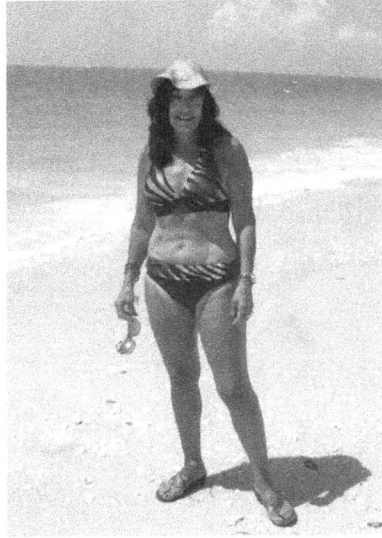

Table of Contents

Why This Book?

When I was a single parent raising four children, working two jobs, attending night classes in an undergraduate degree program and struggling financially, I stumbled upon a book while doing some research in the college library. That book, **Psycho-Cybernetics** by Dr. Maxwell Maltz, changed my life. In fact, the concepts I adopted back then have contributed to my happy, healthy longevity!

Maltz, a plastic surgeon, discovered that it took his patients about 21 days to adjust to their new selves. It didn't matter whether the patient was one who had to acclimate to a surgically enhanced face or one who had to adapt to the loss of a limb. The time span was the same. The brain needs 21 days to develop a new neural pathway.

Yes, I thought. That's what I need, a new pathway! I was under-paid, under-valued, over-worked, and overwhelmed. Hell! I had little to lose. And, all I had to do to start was perform what Maltz referred to as "emotional surgery." Autobiographical note; for me all surgery is emotional. Maltz's self-administered operation required me to do two things:

> First I had to develop an accurate and positive view of myself. At that time, I was so low that I was reaching up trying to find bottom. I had to take a scalpel to myself and excise my self-image as a hopeless loser and adopt a new, dynamic self-image. I had to mimic Maltz's formerly disfigured patients who had to perceive themselves as attractive vs. disfigured. I had to see myself as fully functioning similar to his patients who had lost a limb.

1

Only after I implanted the new me in my mind, could I go on to step two where I had to devise targets: specific, challenging goals.

Maltz's premise: doing these two things activated my brain to function like the computer on a guided missile, designed to automatically find a path to the target.

It worked!

I wrote out five giamongus goals in all the glorious detail of having achieved them. I typed each one on a 5 x 8 card (no computers back then) and listed one action I would take each day for the next three weeks. I didn't achieve my goals in 21 days. However, I did form the habits that allowed me to acquire three degrees, clean up my relationship with my son, start an enormously successful company, and develop a life-long loving relationship with my second husband, Dan. One of my goals, the one I refer to as my anti-aging habit, has resulted in a life-long fitness program that I still follow at 77 years old.

> **My anti-aging goal:** *I am physically, mentally, and psychologically fit. I have the mind, the body, and the energy of a healthy person half my age. I look healthy, I feel healthy, and I am healthy.*

Recent research on how long it takes to form a habit reveals that it could take longer than three weeks to make a lasting change in behavior. More challenging changes are reported to take up to 66 days.

Nevertheless, I cling to Maltz's original assertion. What could be more difficult than adjusting to the loss of a limb?

What I learned and developed over time was my own philosophy toward life and living. *Anti-Aging Habits* is a life-long plan for enjoying a longer, happier, and healthier life.

Just in case you need a nudge to consider reinventing yourself, your outlook, and your life, consider the following:

Every day for the next 19 years, 10,000 baby boomers will turn 65. They want to live their golden years the same way they lived their lives: Changing the way the world works, communicates, and lives. Aging? We ain't gonna take it layin' down!

Then, there is the biggest-ever study of the global burden of disease (GBD2 010) with both good and bad news.

Figure 1. July 2014 Run for Life. 36th consecutive year of winning a medal in my age category.

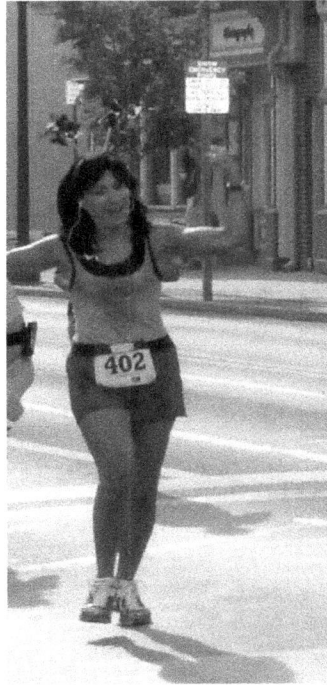

> **The good news**: Over the last four decades, life expectancy around the world has risen dramatically by 11 years for men and 12 years for women.

> **The bad news**: Although we are adding years to our life, we are **not** adding life to our years. In fact, in the two decades prior to 2010, men's life expectancy increased by 4.7 years and women's by 5.1 years—but the extra years of good health were only 3.9 years and 4 years respectively. The primary causes in the gap between the two are physical inactivity and diet (which accounted for 12.5 million deaths).

The best news of all: There are practical, proven, paths for those who want to add years to their life AND life to their years. My research has confirmed that you can form new life-extending and life-enhancing habits in just 21 days. I have spent the past two years conducting research and working with geriatric specialists to identify the exact habits that result in a longer, healthier, more vital, more youthful life span. They are yours in the pages that follow.

The information presented in *Anti-Aging Habits* falls into four broad aspects of longevity: Exercise, Nutrition, Your Brain, and Joyful Living. Although they may not be of equal importance to you based on your current state of fitness, they are all equally important to achieving a longer, livelier life.

Anti-Aging Habits is a journey, more than a map. You do not need to go through it in any particular order. Grow through it vs. go through it. Start where it makes the most sense to you. My hope is that it takes you a long, long, long time.

Having lots of birthdays seems to be the only available way to live a long life.

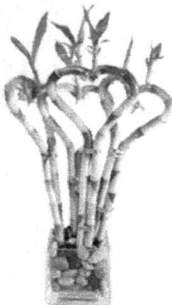

This book is for those of you who want to grow old without aging; who want to look and feel youthful until the day you die, and who want long, healthy, happy lives.

It is for those who, like the bamboo plant – a symbol of longevity, want to be resilient, evergreen, and endure for generations.

You'll find the longevity secrets to resilience, vitality and endurance presented in these five sections.

I. <u>Head Games</u>: How to care for, feed, and train your brain to be smart for life.

II. <u>Food for Life</u>: How to fill your tank with high octane fuel that fires up your engine, fights obesity, and fends off disease.

III. <u>Kick Start your Heart</u>: How to tap into the life-long and long-life benefits of exercise.

IV. <u>The Joy Factor</u>: How to capture the joy of a love affair with life.

V. <u>Fantastic Factoids</u>: Easy to digest summaries of research that will encourage you to sustain your healthy habits and achieve your longevity goals.

Each Chapter closes with "In a Nutshell." Just as the nutritious part of the nut is in the shell, the essence of, or the prime take aways from each chapter, follows in a nutshell.

By adopting the habits recommended in the pages that follow, you can begin to add years to your life and life to your years in just 21 days. As with all change, the best way is **just do it**!

Finally, one of my personal life goals follows:

I share my life experiences, expertise and enthusiasm with others in ways that inspire them to take actions that lead to a happier, healthier, longer life.

Please let me know if I'm on target!

Here's an overview of what you'll find in each section along with a brief summary of each chapter.

Section I. <u>Head Games</u>: How to care for, feed, and train your brain to be smart for life.

Your brain is the most vital organ in the anti-aging process. Nutrition, exercise and social interactions all contribute to a healthy brain. Longevity, the fountain of youth, is your mind. It is the alertness, the vitality, the creativity, and the zeal you bring to your life and the lives of those you know and love. Longevity is your brain on life!

<u>Chapters</u>

1. *No Excuses*

Don't let B. S. [belief systems] limit your youthfulness, liveliness and longevity.

2. *Walk Down a New Street*

How to find the right path, stay on it and avoid the pitfalls.

3. *Train Your Brain*

Three proven ways to retain your memory and mental sharpness.

4. *Get Unblocked*

How unfinished projects, tasks, unresolved interpersonal problems can block energy and enthusiasm, and how to tap into the joy of "completion."

5. *Think Your Way to Longevity*

What happens when the primitive part of your brain perceives peril and how to reframe events to reduce stress, increase energy and save relationships.

6. *Food for Thought*

Eat smart! Consume foods that fuel your brain and fend off cognitive decline.

Section II. <u>Food for Life</u>: How to fill your tank with high octane fuel that fires up your engine, fights obesity, and fends off disease.

The acronym for the Standard American Diet, SAD, says it all! Despite the glut of information about healthy eating, we have higher rates of obesity and chronic disease than ever. We know what to do. So, why don't we eat healthy? One of the reasons may be that our fast-paced, frenetic lives cause us to eat for convenience and speed instead of for nutrition and pleasure. Let's face it, it easier to watch Dr. Oz tell us what to do than actually to change our eating habits.

Your body is the only vehicle you have for traveling through life. Just as you would ruin your engine if you put gasoline in your diesel-fueled car, you'll destroy your body by trying to fuel it with the wrong foods. If you want to be healthy, vital, and energetic, you have to nourish your body with the right fuel.

<u>Chapters</u>

7. *Aging: Defy it with Diet*

How to eat yourself into old age.

8. *Eat Right—Avoid White*

Exclude these foods to live a longer, lighter, livelier life.

9. *Aging is Optional*

How to spice up your diet **and** reduce inflammation with eight foods, herbs and spices.

10. *Drink Up!*

Avoid many of the maladies of aging simply by staying hydrated.

11. *Tips for Tippling*

Know exactly how many ounces of wine, beer, or spirits constitute a "standard drink" and the pay-offs and perils of alcohol.

12. *Get the Perks of Perk*

Drink in longevity with your morning Joe.

Section III. <u>Kick Start your Heart</u>: How to tap into the life-long and long-life benefits of exercise.

Physical inactivity is linked to more than 5 million deaths worldwide per year: More than those caused by smoking. Don't take that lying down! Don't be among the eighty percent (80%) of adult Americans who do not get the recommended amounts of exercise per week. Instead, choose physical activities that are fun, easy to do, and habit forming. Regular exercise not only contributes to a toned, fit body; it keeps your brain sharp!

<u>Chapters</u>

13. *Kick Some Butt*

The how and why of aerobic exercise

14. *Lift the Years Away*

Refuse to lose muscle mass!

15. Mind Your Middle

Reap the many benefits of core training (beyond an awesome six-pack).

16. Stay Limber, Lithe and Lissome

How 10 minutes a day can keep you flexible for life

17. Jump for Life or Skip it

Adopt two of the highest calorie burning activities.

18. Dance and Prance Like Nobody is Watching

Let loose, wiggle your body, and shake your booty!

Section IV. <u>The Joy Factor</u>: How to capture the joy of a love affair with life.

It is not realistic to expect to live your life in a state of bliss. It is reasonable to believe you can transcend many of life's curve balls. You can tap into your innate reservoirs of courage, compassion and gratitude to heighten your sense of wonder and experience more joy and elation as long as you live.

<u>Chapters</u>

19. Lighten Up!

Tap into the joys and benefits of optimism

20. Sex: get it on and get it off!

How getting lucky can contribute to longevity.

21. Unload!

Access the life-extending power of forgiveness.

22. Don't Hesitate—Appreciate!

How an attitude of gratitude contributes to life.

23. Live Life on Purpose

How helping others is the best way to take care of yourself.

24. Think and Act Outside the Box to Stay Outside the Box

How thinking and acting differently can bring joy to others and life to your years.

Section V. <u>Fantastic Factoids</u>: Easy to digest summaries of research that will encourage you to sustain your healthy habits and achieve your longevity goals.

Section I:

Head Games

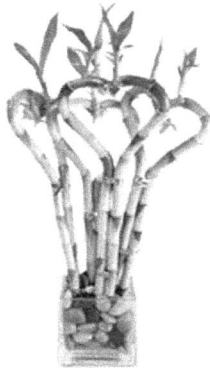

*How to care for, feed, and train your brain
to be smart for life.*

Chapter 1: No Excuses!

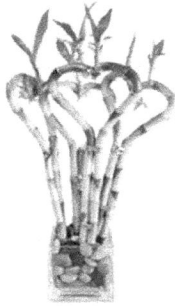

If you don't want to do something,
one excuse is as good as another.
- Yiddish Proverb

The maximum human life-span is 120 years. The greatest deterrent to living that long is our B.S.—our Belief Systems—about longevity. Just a few of which are:

- The belief that genetics is the primary determinant of a long life.

- The conviction that life is a bell-shaped curve—that once we reach a certain plateau, we slide into a mental and physical decline.

- Certainty based on a family member or friend's life, such as *My grandfather drank, smoked, ate red meat, never went to a gym, and he lived to be 90 years old.*

- The conviction that moderation in all you do is the key to longevity.

All of the above is B.S. literally and figuratively!

- Your genetic makeup is NOT the primary influence on longevity. Of the four most significant factors that impact longevity; genes, medical care, lifestyle, and environment, your genetic makeup contributes only 20%. Medical care 10%, and the environment contributes 20% each. Lifestyle has the greatest impact at 50%.

- You can square the curve. According to researchers D. M. Reed, D. J. Foley, L. R. White, H. Heimovitz, C. M. Burchfiel, and K. Masaki reporting in the *American Journal of Health*, failing health in later life is not inevitable. Much of the illness and disability associated with aging is related to modifiable lifestyle factors that are present in middle age. It is never too late adopt new life-supporting habits.

Instead of gradually losing physical and mental capacity, it is possible to maintain your energy, mobility, flexibility, and balance (both physical and mental) until the day you die. Infirmity does not necessarily have to accompany aging.

- Yeah sure, your grandfather or your friend had bad habits. Keep in mind that they are the exception vs. the rule.

- Moderation is the key to deterioration, especially as it relates to physical fitness. Our bones, muscles, cardiovascular system, and brains all need to be stretched to build bone density, muscle strength, keep our blood vessels open, our lung capacity high, our heart muscle robust and to foster neuroplasticity in our brain.

Our B.S. and our comfort zone, the things we know how to do and all of the habits we are used to, limit our youthfulness, liveliness, and longevity. You can move from limiting beliefs and excuses to the you to which you aspire. This book is designed to be your kick in the anatomy: A call to stay conscious of your thoughts and actions and to start now. So…

• Stop smokin', tokin', or otherwise jokin' yourself. Substance abuse will kill your relationships, your love life, your will, and quite possibly your body as well. Give it up! This is not a book on recovery. That is the extent of advice on addiction.

• Avoid the negative and think of yourself as already doing it. Frame your new habits in positive, present tense terms. *I enjoy eating healthy, life-sustaining foods* vs. *I avoid food that is bad for me.* Or, *I look for the positive in all people* vs. *I will stop being critical and judgmental.*

• Don't hesitate to put your heart into your new habits. Be emotional! When planning your new habits think in passionate, motivational terms such as *I love the high I get from daily exercise,* or *I derive joy from volunteering at the childcare center.*

• Don't sabotage yourself by trying to adopt several new habits at once. All you will get is the perfect excuse for non-success. Instead, prioritize. Start with the two or three goals that will have the greatest impact on your life. Focus on moving toward those targets over the next three weeks. Then, identify a few more based on what is important to you.

• All you need to do is embed the achievement of your fondest dreams into your mind in great detail. Spend about ten minutes each day to envision yourself already having attained whatever it is you want to achieve. View yourself enjoying the realization of your goal(s) in minute detail: the colors, the sights, the sounds, and even the smells. Then, take at least one action every day to move yourself toward the goal(s). And, in 21 days, you will have formed a habit.

Here is how it works. Your habits are formed when you repeat certain behaviors or thoughts. In doing so, you create deep and practiced neural pathways. The more you act or think in a certain way the more solid the pathways became. We call them habits. However, just like superhighways, they can be reconstructed or redirected. Your brain is capable of change and you can form new pathways or habits.

In a Nutshell

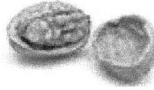

Your genetic makeup is NOT the primary influence on longevity. Your lifestyle has the greatest impact—even more than healthcare and environment.

Poor health in later life is not inevitable. You can make lifestyle changes today that prevent or deter physical and mental decline in later years.

Your body needs to be stretched and strengthened, and your brain challenged in order to keep them fit and agile well into your old age!

You need to be realistic. Addictions harm and can kill your body, mind, and spirit.

You also need to be optimistic. Create positive, detailed mental images of having achieved your goals.

Tap into heart power. Frame your new habits in passionate, emotional terms.

Prioritize. Start with the two or three goals that you desire most. You can set more as you form the life-altering habits necessary to live a longer, livelier, healthier life.

Chapter 2: Walk Down a New Street

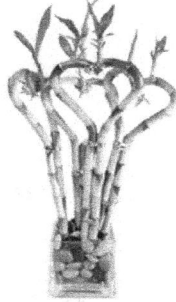

Portia Nelson captured the journey to personal change beautifully in her "Autobiography in Five Short Chapters."

I walk down the street.

There is a deep hole in the sidewalk.

I fall in.

I am lost...I am helpless.

It isn't my fault.

It takes forever to find a way out.

I walk down the same street.

There is a deep hole in the sidewalk.

I pretend I don't see it.

I fall in again.

I can't believe I am in the same place, but,

It isn't my fault.

It still takes a long time to get out.

I walk down the same street.

There is a deep hole in the sidewalk.

I see it is there.

I still fall in…it's a habit.

My eyes are open.

I know where I am.

It is my fault.

I get out immediately.

I walk down the same street.

There is a deep hole in the sidewalk.

I walk around it.

I walk down another street.

Portia Nelson (May 27, 1920 - March 6, 2001) American popular singer, songwriter, actress, and author.

Most of the "holes" that we fall into relative to a long, healthy, lively life are related to:

- Physical inactivity.

- Poor nutrition.

- The belief that we will lose our looks, energy, and vitality.

- Unsatisfactory or limited warm, loving relationships.

- Lack of direction or purpose in life.

- Anticipation of diminished cognition.

- The stress associated with aging.

The chapters that follow recommend evidence-based actions, habits, tools, and techniques to keep you on the new street you chose. Adopt them for 21 days and you will be on the street to a younger, livelier, age-defying you!

Once you've decided to walk down another street, you'll need to do two things to form your new habits.

Step One: Envision the New You

Envision a clear, compelling, picture of the person you want to be. This mental picture will guide your day-to-day actions. So, build it with great detail. For example, if you want to stop feeling tired and drained of energy you might picture yourself in this way:

> *I greet each day with vigor. My enthusiasm sparks my energy that sustains me through the day. Vitality is my natural state whether at work or play.*

Then, take a minute or two to picture yourself exuding that kind of energy while performing your daily activities in great detail. Envision in graphic detail the way you look, act, and feel.

Or, if you want to become more physically fit, you might create a mental picture of yourself in this way:

> *I am at the peak of my physical fitness. I am at my ideal weight; my muscle tone is good and my physical endurance is excellent. I look healthy, I feel healthy, and I am healthy.*

Then, take a minute or two to picture yourself with the body and fitness level to which you aspire. See your lean body, your great pipes, your tight tummy and butt as you walk, jog, bike or lift weights with a beaming big smile on your face. ☺

The more detail and specificity you can build into your mental images, the more likely you will be to achieve the new you. Your new mental images will erase your old mental pictures of yourself as tired, overweight, aging, unloved, aimless, etc., and create new images of yourself in your ideal state.

You get the picture. What you see **really is what you get!** That is because your mind is made up of two parts: your conscious mind and your subconscious mind. The conscious thoughts that you dwell on repeatedly sink into your subconscious mind. Your subconscious mind is like a computer; it can't think on its own. However, it does understand the language of pictures. You paint the picture in your conscious mind, and your subconscious mind adopts it and begins to manifest your vision as a reality.

The first step is to build the image. So, take a few minutes each day to relax and envision your ideal state in exquisite, exciting detail: the sight, feel, smell and sounds of a new you. Create your own personalized YouTube video. Go viral in your own mind—watching yourself in scenes similar to the ones that follow:

- It is easy for me to achieve and maintain my ideal weight of ____. I enjoy eating clean and consume just enough tasty, nutritious foods to adequately fuel my body. At (weight) I feel healthy, I look healthy, and I am healthy.

- I have all the energy I need to accomplish the work of the day and to engage in the leisure activities I love.

- It is easy for me to relate to others in positive ways. I have many warm, close, loving relationships.

- I earn a minimum of $___/year working smart and easy. I invest well, share generously, and spend wisely.

- I enjoy and am good at what I do. I produce worthwhile, high quality, valued goods/services.

- I am at peace with myself, my family and friends, and am happy with my place in the world.

- I am a successful human being. My success does not require me to take advantage of others. I delight in my ability to help others without telling of my good deeds.

- I am at the peak of my physical fitness. I am at my ideal weight; my muscle tone is good and my physical endurance is excellent. I look healthy, I feel healthy, and I am healthy.

- I am a vital, attractive human being.

- I greet each day with a sense of purpose. I pursue my purpose with energy, passion and integrity. I do good and am open to all of the good that comes to me.

- I am a positive, optimistic, happy person.

- I accept and appreciate others for who they are. I find and acknowledge their positive attributes.

- Every day I demonstrate my new habits. I move closer to my ideal self and become more fully functioning, satisfied, and able to enjoy life and all that it has to offer.

Once you take this important first step, your subconscious is geared up and ready to go. You will begin to notice opportunities to achieve the new you that weren't apparent to you before. For instance, you might realize that a reasonably-priced fitness center such as Planet Fitness is within a mile of your home, or that your community offers a variety of fitness classes at times that are convenient for you, or that you really like the taste of "undressed" vegetables. All of those opportunities were there before, but your subconscious wasn't programmed to bring them to your awareness.

Step Two: Take Action

Step two requires you to identify the most important actions you will take (the habits you must form) to get there. What do you need to start doing today and continue doing over the next 21 days so that those actions become second nature? What kinds of new habits will move you toward your dreams?

A few examples of habits that would move you toward the kind of ideal states discussed above follow:

<u>Ideal State</u>: *I greet each day with vigor. My enthusiasm sparks my energy that sustains me through the day. Vitality is my natural state whether at work or play.*

- **Habit: Every day I fuel my body with foods that burn fat and convert to energy** such as fresh fruits and vegetables, lean protein, and calcium-rich low-fat foods. As a result, I have all the energy I need to work and play.

- **Habit: I get a minimum of 7 hours sleep a night.** It feels good to bound out of bed with energy each morning.

- **Habit: I consume no more than one alcoholic drink per day.** Being clear-headed gives me a whole new view of the world.

- **Habit: I drink at least 8 glasses of water a day.** I feel and look refreshed.

<u>Ideal State</u>: *I am at the peak of my physical fitness. I am at my ideal weight; my muscle tone is good and my physical endurance is excellent. I look healthy, I feel healthy, and I am healthy.*

- **Habit: I engage in a minimum of 30 minutes of aerobic exercise six days a week.** I love the high I get from exercise.

- **Habit: I adopt a 20-minute every-other-day weight training program** that focuses on my upper body two days a week and on my lower body two days a week. It feels good to be strong and well-toned.

- **Habit: I eat a healthy diet that consists of 70% fruits, vegetables, and whole grains, 15% lean protein, and 15% unsaturated fats**. My energy is high, my cravings are low, and I'm lookin' damned good!!!

You may have noticed a positive outcome is part of each of the sample habits. There is an excellent reason for identifying the affirmative feelings that will result from your new habits. According to New York Times reporter Charles Duhigg, author of the book *The Power of Habit: Why We Do What We Do in Life and Business*, when you focus on rewards it trains the part of your brain that links positive emotions to new habits, making them easier to adopt and sustain.

The key to adopting new habits is **not** will-power, which requires decision-making and energy to avoid derailment. Instead, habits are formed by reinforcing the behavior you desire with positive rewards! Your habits should **spark** your commitment to achieving your ideal state. Use the spark litmus test to create habits that will change your life.

• **Specific**: State your new habits in specific, concrete terms. *I engage in aerobic exercise 30 minutes a day, 5 days a week* is more likely to move you toward an ideal state than *I start to exercise.*

• **Practice daily**. Whatever you desire; to lose weight, reduce stress, or improve your mental capabilities, you'll need to practice your new habits for 21 days.

• **Align** each habit with a new routine that leads you to engage consistently in a new practice. Charles Duhigg provides several examples of how to do this in his book, *The Power of Habit*. Here is an example: You are stressed at the end of the day. Your current routine is to have a glass of wine. It relaxes you and might even reduce your commitment to avoid snacks. Instead, replace the glass of wine routine with going to the gym. You'll feel better about yourself and train your brain to link the positive emotions associated with more energy and a reduced craving for snacks to your new habit.

- **Realistic**: Take care not to aim for habits that are so challenging that you get overwhelmed or give up. It is ok to start small and ramp up as you go along. Example: *I tell others when I feel as if they are taking advantage of me* is a good beginning if you want to become more assertive vs. *I confront with the skill and ease of a courtroom attorney.*

- **Kudos**: Identify the rewards of your new behaviors. Bask in how good you feel after a good workout, or your smaller size or waistline that comes from good clean eating. Build in ways to celebrate your progress. For example, buy a new pair of slacks after losing 10 pounds or spend a night at the theater with the money you saved from not eating junk food.

Finally, don't keep your planned actions a secret.

Instead, commit at the highest level. There is a hierarchy of new habit formation that goes something like this: Committing to make a change is a good first step. Your chance of success in remembering to do or not do something is enhanced when you write it down. This second level of commitment—writing it down—helps you create a mental picture of success that you can more easily access. Your chance of success is even further improved when you take the time to envision yourself doing it in great detail. The final and highest level of success comes when you speak your commitment to another. At this level, you have put your integrity on the line. Most of us want to live up to our promises!

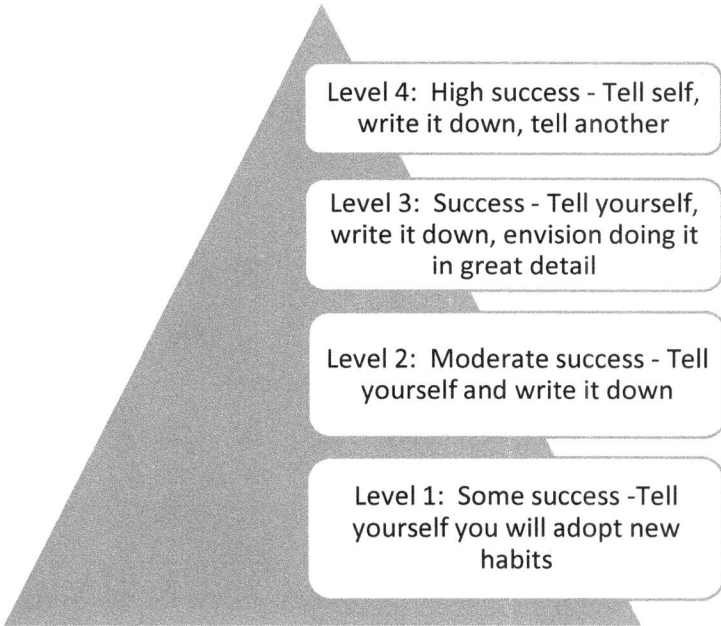

Level 4: High success - Tell self, write it down, tell another

Level 3: Success - Tell yourself, write it down, envision doing it in great detail

Level 2: Moderate success - Tell yourself and write it down

Level 1: Some success -Tell yourself you will adopt new habits

In a Nutshell

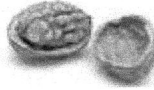

You can start to walk down a new street by taking three important steps:

- Build an exciting, detailed mental picture of the new you and spend a few minutes every day dwelling on that picture.

- Identify the most important actions you will take (the habits you will adopt) to achieve the new you.

- Attach good feelings/rewards to each habit. Rewards, more than will-power, drive the formation of new habits.

-

S P A R K your new habits:

Specific

Practice daily

Align with a new routine

Realistic

Kudos

Commit to your new habits at the highest level: Pledge to adopt them to yourself, write them down, envision yourself doing them, and articulate your commitment to another person.

Chapter 3: Train Your Brain

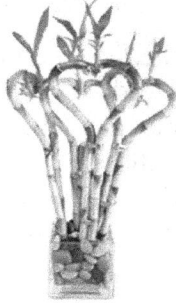

There is a fountain of youth: it is your mind,
your talents, the creativity you bring to your
life, and the lives of people you love. When
you learn to tap this source, you will truly
have defeated age.
- Sophia Loren

Robert Butler, M.D., one of the country's foremost experts on aging, reports that 31% of 65-year-old women are expected to live to age 90 or beyond. Good news, if you can remember it! And, Butler asserts that you can. He writes that people who are having trouble with memory and mental sharpness can—with brain training and increased human interactions—regain as much as two decades of memory. Until recently, it was believed that as we age, our brain's neural networks become fixed, making new learning and cognitive improvement difficult or impossible. Not so! In the past two decades, an enormous amount of research has revealed that our brains never stop adjusting or lose their plasticity, even into very advanced age. Start your brain-training today with a few of these habits:

Habit: Learn something new every day.

One of my dearest friends, Dr. Anthony Ricci, is 99 years old and as sharp as a tack. He does a lot of things right. He eats clean, doesn't smoke, limits alcohol, exercises every day, AND he is curious. He relentlessly studies new and different subjects. Just a few examples: He went to Italy to learn how to make pizza and bread in a brick oven. He came back to the States and built his own oven. His bread is delicious! In addition to learning new recipes, he studies language, religion and history.

Learning is thought to be "neuro-protective." Recent breakthroughs have shown your brain has the lifelong capacity to change and rewire itself (a concept known as neuroplasticity). That response is stimulated when you learn and experience new things. Your brain is able to create new neurons and connections between neurons well into your 90's and beyond. Learning increases connections between neurons, cellular metabolism (the biochemical reactions within cells), and increases the production of nerve growth factor, a substance used by the body to help maintain and repair neurons.

Try it. You'll like it. Learn sign language, bridge, a computer program, a dance, take a class or an on-line course, or do jigsaw, word or number puzzles. Challenge your brain by doing different kinds of puzzles instead of the same type every day. Play computer games: yes! They require speed of processing, a cognitive ability that goes south without regular use. Go to http://www.brainhq.com/# for some great games. Memorize poems, songs, psalms, readings, and lists. The next time you are with a new group of 10 to 20 people, decide to learn all of their names within a given period of time.

Habit: Venture out of your driveway

Go down roads you pass but never travel. Just make sure you have your GPS. The **American Journal of Geriatric Psychiatry** reported the results of a recent study that measured mobility; the degree to which people got around in their environment and how much they see beyond their own home. The study found that people who never leave their home environment during a week were twice as likely to develop Alzheimer's in the five years following the study as those who traveled out of town. People who did not go beyond their driveway or front yard were also more likely to develop mild cognitive disorder.

Habit: Do something silly or outrageous—you are entitled!

You can join me in my quest to liberate myself from the day-to-day activities that get me in a mental rut. Our brains like to be tickled every once in a while. Not only that—others expect older people to act a little bizarre. I meet their expectations and my need to celebrate life by doing the following things which I encourage you to do as well:

- Go to an upscale store not to shop but to "try." I had a blast trying on outrageously expensive fur coats and prom dresses. Try on expensive jewelry, formal wear, or test drive a Porshe convertible.

- Skip. Yes, I mean like you did when you were a kid. I love to skip on the beach and always make a couple of new friends when I do.

- Put a fresh flower in your hair or in a buttonhole.

- Be spontaneous. We were at a local mall recently, listening to a performer who did pretty good impersonations of Frank Sinatra, Bobby Darin, Elvis

Presley, and Tony Bennett. I got up and danced with a five-year- old who was itching to shake it, a lovely woman in a wheelchair, and a delightful man from Ireland. I can't describe how good it made me feel!

• For one day, finish all your sentences with the words "as is written in the book of (insert your name)."

In a Nutshell

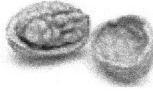

Your brain has a lifelong capacity to change and rewire itself in response to the stimulation of learning and experience.

Learn new things. Doing the same type of puzzle every day is not nearly as effective as continually challenging your brain with new learning—languages, different puzzles, memorization, classes, reading that requires concentration and challenges your thinking, computer games.

Travel. Venture down new paths. You don't have to leave the country (although that works well). Visit different neighborhoods, explore the countryside or the city where you live, take a different route home from the pharmacy or the grocery store.

Tap into the power of silliness. Be immoderate in moderation. Playfulness has been proven to relieve stress, create more balance in life, and to be as revitalizing as a good night's sleep. An occasional burst of outrageousness is wholesome tonic for the brain!

Chapter 4: Get Unblocked

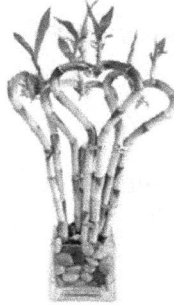

Procrastination is like masturbation.
Sure it feels good at first, but then you
realize you're only screwing yourself.
- Unknown

Constipation and procrastination are inexorably linked. In both conditions you don't give a crap. And, although neither has been reported to make you dead, both cause you to wish you were. At the very least, they can limit the joy of living.

Unlike the other 5 chapters in this section, this one is not supported by research—just my personal experiences. Up until about 20 years ago, it would not have been at all unusual for me to have 15 different projects at some stage of completion. My kids used to accuse me of inventing multitasking. I'm not that way today due to a revelation I had while having a mud bath at a spa in Calistoga Springs, CA.

The purpose of my visit to the spa was to kick back and enjoy a day of pampering. So, I'm in this huge tub, gazing up into a gorgeous blue sky while the attendant shovels about a ton of black, gooey stuff that feels like gritty chocolate pudding all over me. I was supposed to be relaxing. But, all I could think of was my huge "to do" list and why I felt so stalled. Typically a very energetic person, I'd been feeling dragged out, stuck, and joyless. I couldn't seem to make the things that were crucial to me happen. Things like a thesis that was 75% complete, a leadership book that, after three years, was still in the outline stage, a garage in which I couldn't park my car (too full of stuff that needed to be thrown or given away), and an unresolved problem with one of my direct reports. You get the picture. And, at that very moment, I got the picture too! The clouds above the skylight looked just like a funnel.

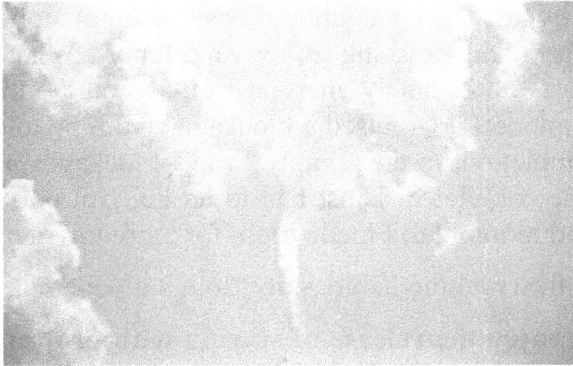

And, all of a sudden, I saw a similar funnel in my head. All my incompletions and partially finished projects were circles crammed into the clouds above the opening of the funnel.

But instead of being neat circular-like pebbles that could pass through, all of my projects were hanging open; incompletions and unfinished tasks were clogging my funnel. No matter how hard I strained, nothing could pass through. Cosmic constipation!!!

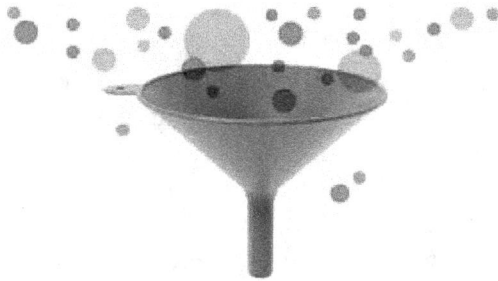

I needed to close the gaps!

I started by attacking a couple of easy incompletions: cleaning out my desk and finishing an overdue report. What a gush of relief. I was immediately energized to take on the thesis. With each completion, I expulsed a blockage. Truth be told, some of the incompletions were simply crap—blockages that didn't need to be completed. I just had to let go. Not only did I feel lighter and more vital; I made room for more joy in my life.

I refer to the resulting habit as my "tough mudder" habit.

Habit: I enjoy the release of staying with projects through to completion. I either finish things or dump them!

In a Nutshell

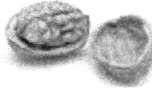

Unfinished projects, business and unresolved interpersonal problems can block your energy, enthusiasm, and joy, causing cosmic constipation.

Unclog your funnel by systematically closing the loops. Finishing a small, easy project can release blockages **and** energy. A small start fuels other completions.

Chapter 5: Think Your Way to Longevity

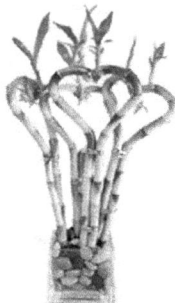

Righteous Indignation: Your own wrath,
as opposed to the shocking bad temper of others.
- Anon

Has another driver ever cut you off in traffic? Or, has someone budged in front of you in a long line?

When adverse events occur, minor or major, they typically trigger three negative emotions; anger (the urge to attack), fear (the urge to escape) and disgust (the urge to expel). These emotions are our primal responses to a perceived threat in our environment—to fight or to run (flight). See table on page 40.

The flight or fight response is responsible, to a significant degree, for your being here today. Thousands of years ago when your ancestors lived in caves, one of them may have found themselves in a situation where they were about to be dinner for a hungry lion. Certainly not a time to stop, reflect and think about it! The fight or flight response allowed that forefather or foremother to live long enough not only get away, but to be around long enough to procreate!

In today's world, the threats we encounter are less apparent and are often perceived or imagined. However, the primitive part of your brain that senses the threat cannot differentiate between a real threat and an imagined or perceived threat. Therefore, it initiates the automatic flight or fight response regardless of threat level. Your body's sympathetic nervous system stimulates your adrenal glands that trigger the release of the potent hormones adrenaline and noradrenaline. Your heart rate and breathing increase and your blood pressure rises. The longer your body stays in this mode, the more damage to your overall health.

Event	What you think	Consequences: Feelings and actions
Someone cuts you off in traffic	<ul><li>What a jerk!</li><li>Where are the police when you need them?</li><li>He/she could have killed me!</li></ul>	<ul><li>Anger</li><li>Speed up and tailgate</li><li>Honk your horn</li><li>Send the universal signal for disgust</li><li>Blood pressure increases</li></ul>
Your significant other complains that you are spending too much time with your friends	<ul><li>That's because he or she has no friends</li><li>He or she is jealous, controlling, selfish, etc.</li><li>He/she doesn't trust me</li></ul>	<ul><li>Disgust</li><li>Frustration</li><li>Lash out</li><li>Stomp out</li><li>Go silent</li><li>Feel resentful</li><li>Stay home and pout</li></ul>
Your doctor reports that the MRI revealed a spot on your kidney	<ul><li>It is probably cancer.</li><li>I'll need major surgery.</li><li>I'm gonna die!</li></ul>	<ul><li>Fear</li><li>Sleepless nights</li><li>Blood pressure increases</li><li>Worry about spouse/kids</li></ul>

The flight or fight response occurs in this manner.

| You experience an event | Your brain fires an emotion | You experience a feeling | And you react |

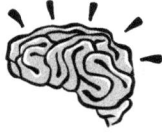

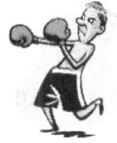

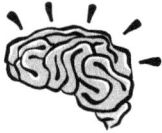

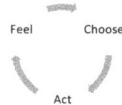

Left unchecked, negative emotions cause hormonal changes that can result in cardiovascular, digestive, and neurological problems. That is because in modern times, fighting (decking your colleague) or fleeing (running away from problems) are not socially acceptable reactions to daily aggravations or even to major crises.

The good news is that in today's world, you can consciously adopt a different response. One that looks like this:

| You experience an event | Your brain responds | You experience a feeling | And you choose how to act |

While we cannot control everything that is going on externally to us, we can control how we respond to it. You can break the flight or fight response by taking a few seconds to think when faced with unpleasant events; reminding yourself that they are not, in themselves, a reason to become angry, fearful or repulsed.

No one can MAKE you feel bad. You have the ability to control your emotional response to external occurrences; to think flexibly and accurately about the causes and implications of such events.

The process is referred to as reframing and is a significant aspect of positive thinking. Reframing is looking at the picture from another perspective. The life events that trouble you can be minor aggravations or major life crises. Your ability to reframe them can reduce stress, increase energy, and save relationships. Looking at the same events from those explored earlier in this chapter, here is how you might reframe them.

Event	What you think	Consequences: feelings and actions
Someone cuts you off in traffic	• He/she was late for work. • He didn't see me. • I'm lucky I was alert.	• Empathy • Increased attention • Relief
Your significant other complains that you are spending too much time with your friends	• He/she misses me when I am gone. • He/she feels neglected. • He/she might want to come along.	• Caring • Dialog to uncover cause of complaints • Positive focus on other
Your doctor reports that the MRI revealed a spot on your kidney	• It may be nothing. • I am relieved it was detected earlier rather than later. • I will be proactive and do things to stay healthy.	• Optimism • A sense of some control over what you can do • Confidence that you can deal with it

It is unfortunate that humans don't come with an owner's manual. The good news is that we can create our own. We can recognize our body's response to events that threaten or stress us and choose how we react. We can actually tell ourselves, "Cool it! This isn't a real threat, calm down."

Positive emotions promote longevity. Positive emotions do more than just help you feel good in the present. New findings, presented at the 2013 symposium at the 25th APS Annual Convention, indicate that positive emotions are associated with healthier gene expression and a more vigorous immune system. This suggests that positive emotions may reduce the physiological "damage" on the cardiovascular system that occurs when you experience negative emotions. In other words, experiencing positive emotions promotes long-term health and increases the likelihood that you will feel good in the future.

My habit: I will always have emotions; I just don't let them have me. I reframe my initial reactions to respond rationally and positively.

In a Nutshell

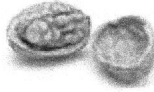

Our initial reactions to unexpected or unwanted situations are a primal response that enabled our ancient ancestors to survive life-threats. The hormones released into our bodies to survive those threats when not released through fighting or fleeing can attack vital organs.

We can moderate our responses to adverse situations by reframing: Thinking accurately and rationally about the event.

Chapter 6: Food for Thought

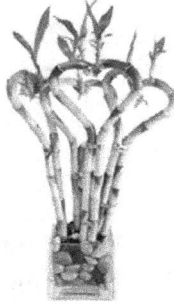

Agassiz does recommend authors to eat fish, because the phosphorus in it makes brains. But I cannot help you to a decision about the amount you need to eat. Perhaps a couple of whales would be enough.
- Mark Twain

Just as food can fuel your body, it can also power your brain and fend off cognitive decline. Eat smart! Adopt this habit.

Habit: Stay Smart by eating the A—B—Sea's & Seeds

A is for antioxidant: Antioxidants protect the brain from the damage of free radicals.

David Perlmutter, M.D., author of ***The Better Brain Book,*** says no part of the body is more sensitive to the damage from free radicals than the brain. Food rich in antioxidants can repair that damage. Good sources of antioxidants include:

- Avocados. Despite the fact that avocado is a fatty fruit, it's a monounsaturated fat, which contributes to healthy blood flow. In addition to being an antioxidant, avocados can lower blood pressure. Hypertension (or high blood pressure) is a risk factor associated with a decline in cognitive abilities. Since avocados are high in calories, limit consumption to 1/4 to 1/2 of an avocado a day.

• Pomegranates or pomegranate juice. You can gain the anti-oxidant benefits with about 2 oz./day.

• Citrus fruits and colorful vegetables.

• Dark chocolate is an excellent source of antioxidants which is a good news/bad news story. The good news is that chocolate stimulates the production of endorphins which help improve your mood. The bad news is that you don't need much to get the benefits. A half ounce a day will provide all the advantages you need.

B is for brain-boosting foods:

• Beans provide your brain with a steady stream of energy in the form of glucose. All beans are good for your brain. My favorites are lentil, kidney and black soy beans.

• Brewed Tea: 2 or 3 cups of freshly brewed tea a day provide antioxidants as well as boost brain power by enhancing memory, focus and mood.

• Blueberries: Steven Pratt, M.D., calls them "Brainberries." Some research indicates that blueberries help protect the brain from oxidative stress and may even reduce the effects of Alzheimer's and dementia. Aim for at least one cup of fresh or frozen blueberries a day.

•   Brown grains and brown rice: Whole grains, such as steel-cut oats, whole-grain breads, and brown rice can reduce the risk of cognitive decline because they promote good blood flow to your entire organ system including your brain. Although wheat germ is not technically a whole grain, it provides similar benefits.

Sea's & Seeds:

•   Deep-water fish, such as salmon, and oily fish such as sardines and herring are rich in omega-3 fatty acids, which are essential for brain function. They also have anti-inflammatory benefits. I eat 3 to 4 oz. of salmon, steelhead trout, or yellowfin tuna at least 3 times a week.

•   Seeds and nuts are reported to lessen cognitive decline due to their high levels of vitamin E. You can get the brain benefits of seeds and nuts with only one ounce a day of any of the following: walnuts, hazelnuts, Brazil nuts, filberts, almonds, cashews, peanuts, sunflower seeds, sesame seeds, flax seed, and non-hydrogenated nut butters such as peanut butter, almond butter, and tahini. It is best to eat unsalted nuts either raw or roasted.

In a Nutshell

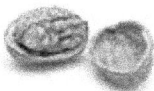

Nuts to you! Nuts are great brain boosters along with other great tasting foods that include dark chocolate, avocados, and blueberries. Other smart foods are cold water fish, herring, sardines, pomegranates, colorful vegetables, whole grains, whole-grain bread, and beans. Wash it all down with a cup of freshly brewed tea.

Section II:

Food for Life

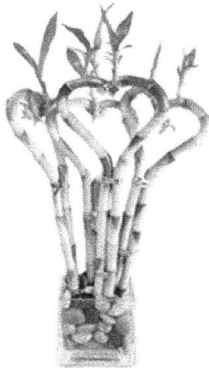

How to fill your tank with high octane fuel that fires up your engine, fights obesity, and fends off disease.

Chapter 7: Aging—Defy it with Diet

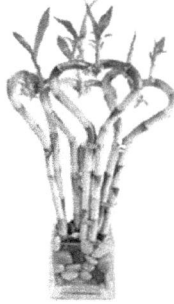

Life is too short not to eat healthy
and it's even shorter if you don't.

A quick search on Amazon reveals that there are nearly 120,000 books on nutrition or diet. I am not going to add to the glut (pun intended). You can't eat literature; it's very dry and not at all nutritious.

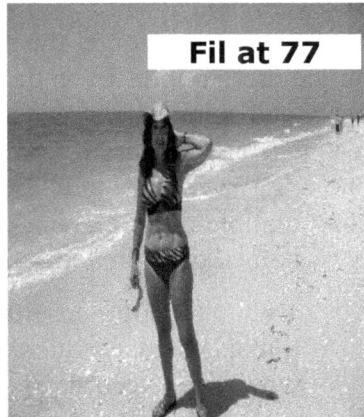

Fil at 77

Instead, I would like to share two important aspects of nutrition and longevity. The first is the mortal danger of common dietary habits. The second is easy-to-follow nutritional advice that has enabled me to achieve and maintain my ideal weight and a high level of energy and good health well into my 70's.

Danger! The typical American diet is a killer

The typical American diet contributes to Metabolic Syndrome, a condition that puts you at major risk for diabetes and heart disease. If you have at least three of the following conditions, you have Metabolic Syndrome:

- A resting blood pressure of 130/85 or higher (either number), or you're currently taking blood-pressure-lowering medications.

- A waist circumference of greater than 35 inches in women and greater than 40 inches in men.

- An HDL (good cholesterol) level of less than 40 mg/dL in men and less than 50 mg/dL in women, or you're currently taking HDL-raising meds.

- A fasting triglyceride level of 150 mg/dL or higher or you're currently taking triglyceride-lowering medications.

- A fasting blood glucose level of 100 mg/dL or higher.

Many people try to get their weight to a healthy level by going on the diet du jour. Even though most diet fads last longer than a day and some have great staying power, they generally do not result in permanent weight loss. This is because they require one or more of the 3 P's: pre-packaged foods, point computation, or permanent calorie planning, none of which can be sustained over the long-term because:

- People lose the patience and the persistence that it takes to constantly count, compute and tally every morsel. According to the late Jackie Gleason, "the second day of a day of a diet is always easier than the first. By the second day you are off it."

- Tiny portions are not satisfying and often result in binging.

- There is a lack of variety in pre-packaged meals.

The alternative is to form a habit similar to the one that follows.

Habit: Shed extra pounds by eating the right foods 5 or 6 times a day to ensure you are never hungry.

Then, adopt an **easy two-pronged approach to good nutrition.**

Prong 1: I used to diet on anything I could lay my hands on. Now I avoid going on diets. Instead, I've adopted the 70-15-15 life-long nutritional plan. I fuel my body in this way:

- 70% of my calories come from plant-based foods: Fruits, vegetables, and whole grains.

- 15% of my calories come from protein: Fat-free dairy products, fish, poultry, and (rarely) lean meat. Most people can get all the protein their bodies need in a 1/2 cup of non-fat cottage cheese or a piece of fish, poultry, or lean meat that is the size of a deck of cards.

- 15% of my calories come from healthy fats: polyunsaturated and monounsaturated fats.

Polyunsaturated fats are those with two essential fatty acids, Omega-6 and Omega-3, which come from foods such as sunflower seeds, avocados, walnuts in their natural state (skip the shells), olive oil, soybeans, tofu, flaxseed, and fatty fish such as salmon, tuna, mackerel, and trout. Some other sources of "good fats" include olives, sunflower oil, peanuts, peanut butter, peanut oil, almonds, macadamia nuts, hazelnuts, pecans, cashews. Your body requires these fatty acids to keep you alive and well, **but** it cannot produce them on its own. You must supply a sufficient amount through diet.

Monounsaturated fat is another good fat. Research shows that monounsaturated fats may help lower your bad (LDL) cholesterol levels, which means a diet containing a sufficient amount of monounsaturated fat may actually help reduce your risk of heart disease and stroke. Monounsaturated fats are most abundant in foods like nuts and various plant oils such as olive oil and canola oil.

Warning!!!! All fats are high in calories. So, even though poly- and monounsaturated fats are "good fats" it isn't wise to consume vast quantities. Five to ten nuts a day is ok.

Some good news about fat: a Swedish study published in the journal, *Stroke* (a deadly name for any publication!), that tracked the diets of 75,000 men and women over a decade found that those who ate the most low-fat dairy foods and beverages were 12% less likely to have a stroke. Experts report that this is because low levels of Vitamin D increase your risk of stroke. Low-fat dairy products, such as skim milk, low-fat yogurt, and cottage cheese are fortified with vitamin D.

So, what does the 70-15-15 life-long eating plan look like in terms of a typical day?

Breakfast

- One cup of steel-cut oats. Cooked cereals are a better choice than dry cereals because they are less calorie dense and more filling.

- A bowl of mixed fruit: 1/2 banana, 2 or 3 kinds of melon, strawberries and blueberries, topped with ½ cup of fat-free, no-salt-added cottage cheese.

Mid-morning Snack

- Cup of low sodium meatless soup or an apple or pear or handful of baby carrots and celery.

Lunch

- Large mixed vegetable salad topped with sunflower seeds or walnuts with balsamic glaze or balsamic vinegar and a teaspoon of olive oil.

Mid-afternoon Snack

- Same as mid-morning snack.

Dinner

- ¼ lb. baked or broiled chicken tenders, or fish.

- ¾ cup brown rice, or whole-wheat pasta, or medium baked potato.

- 1 cup mixed vegetables.

- Small green salad.

- Jell-O or cup of fat-free, no-sugar-added ice cream or frozen yogurt.

Just one of the many benefits of adopting the 70-15-15 eating plan and eating 5-6 times a day is that you will not be hungry after dinner. If you want to lower or maintain your current weight, it is a lot easier to do so if you **don't eat after dark**.

Prong 2: Know what foods to avoid and what foods you can eat until you are full without adding to your calorie intake.

Careful food choices and restricting calories have been credited with extending life. According to Italian researchers, the protein CREB1 is triggered by a calorie restricted diet and activates genes linked to longevity and to the proper functioning of the brain. Calorie restriction is defined as eating

25 to 30 percent less than normal while maintaining optimal nutrition. Some easy, healthy ways to reduce calorie consumption follow.

- **Eat these foods until you are full**: Carrots, celery, all forms of lettuce, peppers, squash, zucchini, tomatoes, cabbage, and most fruits and vegetables. The nutritional value of these foods remains the same whether you eat them cooked or raw.

- **Avoid calorie dense foods**. Calorie dense foods are those that contain a lot of calories for their portion size. Think a tiny piece of cheesecake or a small portion of French fries (naughty!!!). You can separate calorie dense foods into three categories:

The good: Potatoes, whole-wheat pasta, whole-grain breads, rice (not white), and fruit juice (although your body prefers the fruit vs. the juice). Oils, nut butters, nuts, avocados, and bananas are calorie dense as well, but good for you in **small quantities** because they provide necessary vitamins and minerals.

The ok: Lean meats, low-fat cheeses, and over-the-counter protein supplements (your body prefers protein from food vs. drinks and powders), and pizza. Small amounts of the ok foods can contribute to good health. And, don't despair! Pizza can be healthy if it is made with whole wheat dough, low in sodium, and topped with lots of veggies and an itty, bitty sprinkling of cheese.

The bad: Trans fats (products that have hydrogenated oil as an ingredient) and saturated fats (come primarily from animal sources) such as meat, lard, butter and cheese. Calorie dense foods with little or no nutritional value including fried foods, chips, crackers, cheesecake, candy and candy bars, donuts, danish, sugary cereals, cake, most baked goods, ice cream and puddings. Oh, and don't forget bread and rolls dipped in olive oil and grated cheese (as bad as a piece of cheesecake).

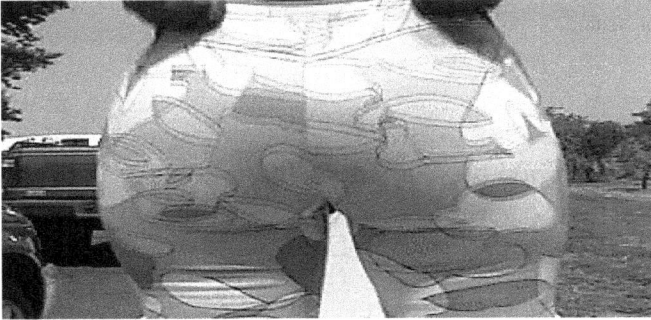

Rich, fatty foods are like destiny: They too, shape our ends.

In a Nutshell

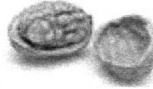

Follow the nutritional advice in this chapter to maintain a healthy weight **and** to avoid developing age-related diseases such as high blood pressure, high cholesterol, cancer, and heart disease.

Eat 5 or 6 times a day. Include a plentiful variety of fruits and vegetables.

Avoid saturated fats and trans fats.

Limit your consumption of red meat and full-fat dairy products, and increase lean protein, omega 3-fatty acids such as cold-water fish, and plant protein such as beans and walnuts.

Chapter 8: Eat Right—Avoid White

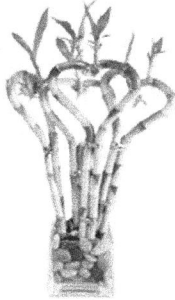

*Statistics show that of those who contract
the habit of eating, very few survive.*
- George Bernard Shaw

Crossing the white line while driving can halt aging—permanently! Crossing the white food line can be equally as dangerous. If you can avoid just three white foods your life ride will be longer, lighter and less dangerous. Let's start with the most ubiquitous white danger:

> • **Salt**. For years, doctors have been saying a diet high in salt is bad for your heart. When you eat **too much** salt, which contains sodium, your body holds extra water to "wash" the salt from your body. In some people, this may cause blood pressure to rise. The added water puts stress on your heart and blood vessels. Recent research indicates that it is REALLY dangerous for women's hearts! *Hypertension Magazine* cited an 11-year study of over 9,000 adults that found women who had a 15 point rise in systolic blood pressure

increased their odds of cardiovascular disease by 56% compared to a 32% increase for men. Research links salt to cancer, diabetes, dementia, and kidney disease. And, if that is not enough to scare the salt out of you, this will: sodium can also make you fat. Brain scans show that sodium triggers dopamine, the feel-good neurotransmitter. So, the more salt you eat, the more you want. Sodium also boosts insulin production, which leads to weight gain.

Surprisingly, Americans' sodium intake breaks down like this according to the FDA, US Food and Drug Administration.

    o   77% from packaged and restaurant food.

    o   12% naturally occurs in foods that include beets, celery, carrots, spinach and chard.

    o   11% is added to food while cooking or at the table.

Less than one-quarter of your sodium intake comes from the salt shaker! And, more than 75% is in processed foods. To avoid curves and cardio problems aim to keep your sodium intake below 1500 mg a day. An excellent resource for keeping your sodium low is the Salt Solution Program published by *Prevention Magazine.*

Another excellent eating plan is the DASH diet, developed by the National Heart, Lung and Blood Institute to help people prevent and treat high blood pressure. The DASH approach to reducing sodium intake emphasizes eating lots of fruits, vegetables, whole grains and low-fat dairy substitutes. *U.S. News & World Report* cites it as #1 on its annual list of best diet plans.

(*Important note:* Despite a May 2013 Institute of Medicine report that concluded there is insufficient evidence for the health benefits of reducing sodium below 2,300 mg, the American Heart Association, as well as many experts, have suggested that people should aim for no more than 1,500 mg of sodium per day. The 1,500 mg level is recommended for older adults, hypertensives, and blacks who are particularly vulnerable to the effects of high sodium intake.)

• Refined **sugar** is another deterrent to liveliness and longevity! Refined sugar has been described as lethal because it provides "empty" calories. It lacks the natural minerals present in sugar beet or cane. Refined sugar is worse than natural sugar because its digestion, detoxification, and elimination drain and leach your body of precious vitamins and minerals. Excess sugar is stored in your liver in the form of glucose (glycogen) which makes your liver expand like a balloon. When your liver is filled to capacity, the excess glycogen is returned to your blood in the form of fatty acids which are transported to every part of your body and stored in the most inactive areas: The belly, the buttocks, the breasts, and the thighs. Then—and here is the frightening part—when those places are filled, the fatty acids go to your organs, such as your heart and kidneys, where they slow them down and cause organ tissue to degenerate. According to the American Heart Association, women should not consume more than 6 teaspoons of added sugar (sweeteners and syrups that are added to foods in processing or at home) a day and men shouldn't consume more than 9 teaspoons a day. These guidelines don't apply to natural sugars such as those found in fruits, vegetables, or dairy products.

•   The third **white** is refined **flour**. It has been said that "white bread is dead bread." That's because the flour used to make white bread is chemically bleached. So when you eat white bread, you are also eating residual chemical bleach. The process of making flour white removes half of the healthy unsaturated fatty acids, that are high in food value. Also, virtually all vitamin E is lost with the removal of the wheat germ and bran. Between 50 and 95% of all other nutrients such as calcium, phosphorus, magnesium, manganese, potassium, copper, thiamin, riboflavin, and niacin are lost as well.

Refined flour is a simple carbohydrate which enters the bloodstream rapidly. This tricks your pancreas into releasing too much insulin, which causes a drop in your blood sugar which can cause you to feel lethargic, mentally confused, weak, and hungry. Refined flour causes weight gain because it alters your metabolism. According to the U.S. Department of Health, if two groups of people take in the same number of calories, but one group gets its calories from refined products, while the other group consumes calories in the form of whole grains (such as bulgar, whole wheat, and brown rice), fruits, nuts and vegetables; the refined products group will gain weight, while the other will not. One of the best ways to limit refined flour is to read the labels of packaged food products. Not just the front label — where it may proclaim "whole wheat" or "natural" — but the ingredient list which is usually on the back or side of the package. If "enriched flour" is the first ingredient listed, avoid it!

As you may recall, I don't eat meat or other fatty foods. Nevertheless, I started this year with 15 extra pounds. With only three changes to my diet, reducing my salt intake to less than 1,500 mg a day, and avoiding refined sugar and refined flour, I was able to lose 15 lbs in 4 months. And, my weight remains steady at my ideal lifetime weight of 125 lbs.

Afraid that you've already fallen prey to the whites and recognize that you need to shed some pounds? Watching your white intake is a good start. When you combine it with the coming chapters, you'll be a lean, mean energy machine. In Chapter 13, "Kick Some Butt" you'll see that I exercise aerobically an hour a day and you can develop habits that will allow you to do the same. Chapter 14 details my easy-to-do every-other-day weight training. And Chapter 15 describes a basic, yet essential, series of core exercises.

In a Nutshell

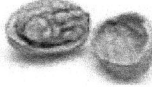

Avoid refined and processed foods. Don't cross the white line. Limit refined flour, refined sugar, and salt. Instead, consume whole grains such as brown rice and bulgar.

Chapter 9: Aging is Optional

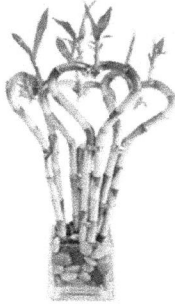

Pogo was right: "We have met the enemy and it is us!"

Aging is something we create in our own bodies. It is the side effect of inflammation.

Inflammation is a good news/bad news story. The good news: inflammation is your body's way of protecting you against infectious disease. Think. You get a small cut on your finger. It gets red and swollen. Inflammation forming around the wound wipes out damaged tissue, kills any unwanted bacteria, and helps you heal. Inflammation occurs in anticipation of something malevolent.

Here is the bad news. Everyday modern living can trigger the inflammatory response in your body. Emotional stress, poor diet, lack of exercise, exposure to toxins, chemicals, and air pollution can turn your immune system into a big bully eager to pummel anything and penetrate your every last cell.

Russell Tracy, a professor of pathology and biochemistry at the University of Vermont College of Medicine, reports that inflammation predicts heart attacks, heart failure, becoming diabetic, frailty in old age, cognitive function decline, and even cancer to a certain extent. Inflammation, the very weapon your immune system uses to fight the diseases of aging, contributes to aging! We are, indeed, our own worst enemy!

Although there is no conclusive proof that inflammation is the root cause of aging, there is enough evidence that reducing it offers an unparalleled opportunity for a longer, healthier life.

My grandfather used to say, "better to spend money on food than on doctors." A good motto for a man who was one of the original chain-store grocers! Grandpop Pietro lived in an age when shoppers couldn't purchase dinner in a box, a tin foil pan, or a plastic bag. Grandmom Grace and the other homemakers of her time prepared meals from scratch and added spices for variety. My grandparents and their progeny benefitted greatly. My mom and her seven siblings lived well into their 90's. But, I digress. Back to how to reduce inflammation.

Today's scientists have begun to believe that aging is a disease. They have discovered many foods, herbs, and spices that can deter or prevent inflammation. I prefer to think they, and Grandpop Pietro, are right.

My anti-aging, anti-inflammatory habit: It is easy for me to eat an anti-aging diet. I spice up wholesome foods with anti-inflammatory herbs and spices.

Seven spices that have been shown to pack a powerful punch to the inflammation bully are:

- Cinnamon. Lab studies confirm that cinnamon may reduce inflammation, have antioxidant effects, and fight bacteria. According to Dr. David Heber, world-renowned nutritionist, cinnamon has additional health benefits. It is rich in polyphenols—natural substances that appear to act like insulin in the body. Polyphenols may help regulate blood sugar levels.

Dr. Richard A. Anderson, of the U.S. Agriculture Department's Beltsville Human Nutrition Research Center, has shown that sprinkling the equivalent of one-quarter to one-half a teaspoon of cinnamon (on cereal or fruit, for example) twice a day lowers glucose, cholesterol, and triglyceride levels by up to 30%. A promising payoff for people at risk for diabetes and heart disease.

• Chili Peppers. Some like it hot and that is a good thing! Hot peppers (like chili and cayenne) are rich in capsaicin, a chemical that's used in topical creams that reduce pain and inflammation. There is an added benefit to consuming chili peppers. Research suggests that three chili peppers a day could boost calorie burn after a meal by 40 to 100 calories. Hot stuff!

• Ginger. I remember my mother giving me a glass of ginger ale for an upset stomach. Now I know why. One of its active ingredients, gingerol, is effective against nausea and pain, plus it inhibits an enzyme that causes inflammation.

• Oregano contains a compound, rosmarinic acid, that is both a potent germ-killer and a powerful antioxidant. Oregano is believed to be one of the greatest anti-oxidant foods.

• Parsley. In addition to its anti-inflammatory properties, parsley is rich in many vital vitamins, including vitamins C, B 12, K and A. Parsley keeps your immune system strong, tones your bones and heals the nervous system. Parsley, not to be dismissed as a pretty little garnish, contains apigenin which makes your blood platelets less sticky and less likely to form clots that cause heart attacks.

- Turmeric. Not only has the curcumin in turmeric been proven to have beneficial effects on the immune function of people with diabetes, preliminary studies indicate that it may help prevent the development of the brain plaques associated with Alzheimer's.

- Thyme. In Ancient Egypt thyme was used for embalming, so we know it keeps you dead. Modern day research indicates that it can keep us alive as well. Take your thyme! Its antioxidant phenols and flavonoids protect DNA against oxidative damage.

Jerry Saltz, columnist for *New York Magazine*, once said, "The secret of food lies in memory—of thinking and then knowing what the taste of cinnamon or steak is." I think it is the other way around: The secret of memory lies in food.

Please take this information to heart. Not only because anti-inflammatory recommendations can prevent heart disease but because MOST diseases have an underlying etiology involving inflammation. Conditions such as Alzheimer's, allergies, arthritis, asthma, cancer, diabetes, heart disease, and inflammatory bowel disorders can be aggravated or made better depending on your diet.

Variety may be the spice of life. But spice makes life taste better and last longer.

In a Nutshell

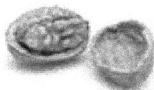

Spice it up with anti-inflammatory herbs and spices.

Follow the dietary advice in Chapter 7, Aging—Defy it with Diet. Eat plenty of fruits and vegetables. Minimize saturated and trans fats and partially hydrogenated oils. Eat a good source of omega-3 fatty acids, such as fish or fish oil supplements, and walnuts. Limit your protein sources to chicken and low or non-fat dairy foods. Limit red meat.

Minimize your intake of the three whites (salt, enriched flour and sugar) as recommended in Chapter 8, Eat Right—Avoid White. Instead, eat whole grains such as brown rice and bulgur wheat.

Avoid refined foods and processed foods. See Chapter 8.

Chapter 10: Drink Up!

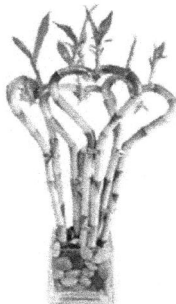

In wine there is wisdom, in beer there is freedom,
in water there is bacteria.
- Benjamin Franklin

Habit: I enjoy drinking 64 ounces of water every day.

It was difficult for me to form this habit. Maybe that is because I have been unconsciously channeling Ben Franklin! More likely it is because I can recall only a few instances in my entire life when I have felt thirsty. This is downright frightening because as we age, the less water we consume, the less we want to drink. In a fair and equitable world this would apply to alcohol as well! Nevertheless, when we don't drink enough water, we risk dehydration and other serious health problems.

Some facts that have helped me form my water habit:

- Seniors tend to get confused over the difference between hunger and thirst. I've found that when I have a hankering for food, it is often a signal of thirst. So, I drink a glass of water. Even when it doesn't assuage my hunger, it contributes to my 64 ounces a day.

• A Virginia Tech study indicates that drinking water before a meal enhances weight loss.

• I carry a bottle of water with me when I jog. I drink just to reduce the weight of the bottle.

• An empty glass on the top of my coffee maker is my reminder to drink 10 ounces as soon as I get up in the morning.

Seven proven facts have influenced me to drink more water as well. Things like:

> 1.   Our brains are about 85% water. Water is fuel for the brain. It provides your brain with the electrical energy necessary for thinking and memory. According to Dr. Corinne Allen, founder of the Advanced Learning and Development Institute, brain cells need twice the energy of our other cells. Our brains depend on proper hydration to function optimally. Brain cells require a delicate balance between water and various elements to operate, and when you don't drink enough water, that balance is disrupted. Your brain cells lose efficiency. When your brain is getting enough water, you think faster, more clearly and are more focused. Dehydration can impair short-term memory and the recall of long-term memory. Symptoms of dehydration, which can cause death in extreme circumstances, include confusion, drowsiness, labored speech, dry mouth, and sunken eyeballs (not to be confused with a severe hangover).

2.   You even lose water while sleeping. Even if you don't sweat it, or don't get up to pee, you expel moisture with every breath. So a good night's sleep can dry you out.

3.   Staying well-hydrated can reduce the risk of dementia, Alzheimer's and Parkinson's.

4.   When your brain is fully hydrated, you enjoy better concentration and alertness.

5.   Side effects for seniors who do not drink enough water extend far beyond dehydration and can include arthritis, sore muscles, dry skin, digestive problems and constipation.

6.   Water is a lubricant. It greases your joints, regulates temperature, and moistens the lungs to allow for easy breathing.

7.   Kidney function is dependent on adequate water. To stay healthy, your kidneys must excrete a minimum of ten ounces of waste per day. When water is not available, there is nothing to dissolve your body's waste products (uric acid and urea). As a result, those waste products build up and lead to kidney stones, while putting additional strain on your kidneys to find adequate liquid to expel the toxins.

Millions of people have lived long, healthy lives without coffee or alcohol (I can't imagine), but not one person is reported to have lived without water.

In a Nutshell

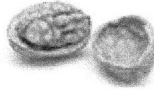

Drink 64 ounces of water a day.

We often confuse hunger with thirst. Drinking lots of water can contribute to weight loss.

When your brain is getting enough water, you think faster, more clearly, and are more focused.

Staying well-hydrated can reduce the risk of dementia, Alzheimer's, and Parkinson's.

Inadequate water consumption can contribute to dehydration, kidney disease, difficulty breathing, joint pain, arthritis, sore muscles, dry skin, digestive problems, and constipation.

Chapter 11: Tips for Tippling

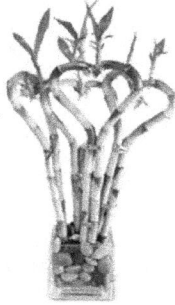

The University of Nebraska says that elderly people that drink beer or wine at least four times a week have the highest bone density. They need it—they're the ones falling down the most.
-Jay Leno

Alcohol consumption is one of the few activities in life where there is no reward, and could possibly result in a penalty, for exceeding the standard. So, let's begin by defining a standard drink. A standard drink is 0.6 ounces of pure alcohol which translates to:

12 oz. of beer

8 oz. of malt liquor

.5 oz. of wine

1.5 oz. of 80 proof distilled spirits (brandy, whiskey, rum, vodka or gin)

For those of you wondering *how many standard drinks I can have a day without risk to my health,* there is no one definition for safe levels of alcohol consumption.

However, there are Dietary Guidelines for Americans Services issued by the US Departments of Agriculture and Health & Human. Low-risk drinking is:

- No more than 1 standard drink per day for women

- No more than 2 standard drinks per day for men

Warning: This is not intended to serve as an average over several days, nor is it advisable to consume your one-week allocation all at one sitting (or falling down).

Alcohol does have some health benefits. However, it may also cause health risks. My advice is to examine both the benefits and risks before forming a habit.

First the benefits:

- The good news about booze is that some studies suggest that red wine may help decrease the chance of developing atherosclerosis, a disease that causes plaque buildup in your arteries. The source of that benefit is the antioxidant in red wine called resveratrol, which may help prevent heart disease by increasing the good cholesterol in a person's body. Since I am not fond of red wine, I take resveratrol in tablet form (from GNC).

- Moderate alcohol consumption could:

    o Reduce your risk of dying from a heart attack.

    o Possibly reduce your risk of strokes, particularly ischemic strokes.

     o   Lower your risk of gallstones.

     o   Possibly reduce your risk of diabetes.

The risks:

Before you begin celebrating the good news, here are some additional findings:

- Light to moderate drinking (one drink a day for women and two for men) can increase the risk of breast, colon, oral, liver, and esophageal cancers. The research, reported in the *British Medical Journal*, was based on a review of 136,000 men and women who were studied for 30 years. According to scientists at Harvard T.H. Chan School of Public Health and Brigham and Women's Hospital, those who drank more showed an even higher risk of alcohol-related cancers.

- New research from UCSF Medical Center has established a strong causal link between alcohol consumption and a dangerous form of heart palpitation. People with atrial fibrillation had nearly 4.5 times greater chance of an episode when they consumed alcohol.

- Heavy drinking, including binge drinking, can cause serious health problems, including:

     o   Certain cancers, including breast cancer and cancers of the mouth, pharynx, larynx, esophagus, and liver.

     o   Pancreatitis.

     o   Sudden death if you already have cardiovascular disease.

     o   Heart muscle damage (alcoholic cardiomyopathy) leading to heart failure.

- o   Stroke.
- o   High blood pressure.
- o   Cirrhosis of the liver.
- o   Suicide.
- o   Accidental serious injury or death.

Given what I know about alcohol, I drink responsibly and in moderation. My healthy habit is simply:

Habit: I can relax, have fun, enjoy good company, and a good meal equally as well with or without alcohol. I enjoy an occasional drink.

In a Nutshell

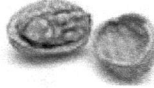

If you don't drink, don't drive yourself to start. Even though there are some health benefits associated with moderate alcohol consumption, the health risks of excessive alcohol consumption far outweigh the benefits of a few drinks a week.

Chapter 12: Get the Perks of Perk

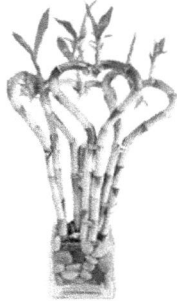

You should stop drinking coffee only if your Doctor
tells you your blood type is Folgers.
- Unknown

I did not have to form a coffee habit. I love coffee! Just not as much as many senior citizens who, according to ***SeniorJournal.com***, would rather give up sex than stop drinking coffee! The study was reported in 2004, and I have been unable to find references as to who conducted it, where it was done, and how many subjects were involved. According to recent research about the longevity benefits of coffee, many of those survey participants should still be alive and kicking. If they are, they are not talking because I cannot find such an unlikely claim validated by a healthy, happy octogenarian!

There are 10,000 baby boomers turning 65 every day, many of whom I have known personally. It is inconceivable to me that any one of them would give up sex before coffee. My research sample is small (me and my friends). So, I'll let it go and move on to the benefits of coffee.

• Research from the National Cancer Institute and AARP says that senior citizens who drink coffee, caffeinated or decaffeinated, have a lower risk of death. Neal Freedman, Ph.D., Division of Cancer Epidemiology and Genetics, NCI, and his colleagues examined the association between coffee drinking and risk of death in 400,000 U.S. men and women ages 50 to 71 who participated in the NIH-AARP Diet and Health Study. Participants were followed from 1955 until they died or December 2008 (whichever came first). The study revealed a correlation between a reduced risk of death and the amount of coffee consumed. Those who drank three or more cups of coffee a day had a 10% lower risk of death. I can live with that!

• More java good news: Coffee has been found to reduce the risk of depression in senior citizens. Michel Lucas, Ph.D., R.D., from the Harvard School of Public Health, Boston, conducted a 10-year study of 50,739 U.S. women with an average age of 63. Participants had no depression at the start of the study in 1996 and were followed up with through June 2006. The study looked at the impact of caffeinated coffee consumption and the risk for depression. The findings:

o Those who consumed two to three cups of coffee per day had a 15 percent decrease in relative risk for depression.

o Those consuming four cups or more per day had a 20 percent decrease in relative risk.

- Studies indicate that men who drink coffee have a lower risk of prostate cancer and women coffee drinkers have less risk of breast cancer.

- A 2012 report in The Archives of Internal Medicine indicates that coffee drinking may lower the risk of Parkinson's disease, type 2 diabetes, liver cancer, and cirrhosis.

- Drinking between three and five cups of coffee a day could cut the chance of developing Alzheimer's disease by up to 20 percent, according to a report published by the Institute for Scientific Information on Coffee.

I don't know how people live without coffee,
I really don't.
- Martha Quinn

In a Nutshell

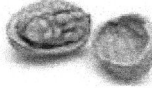

Three to five cups of coffee per day can reduce the risk of the 3 D's: dementia, depression, and death.

Section III:
Kick Start Your Heart

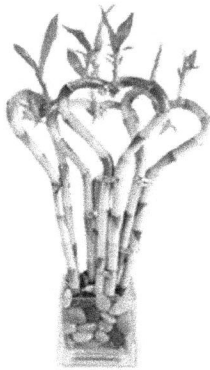

How to tap into the life-long
and long-life benefits of exercise.

Chapter 13: Kick Some Butt!

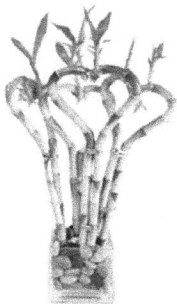

A sweet life is a sweaty life.
- Toni Sorenson

There is nothing like a "death threat" to get someone to change self-defeating habits. One day when my husband, Dan, was in his early forties, he gave up smoking and never smoked again. All it took was a major coronary blockage followed by advice from his cardiologist; *if you want to die, keep smoking.* So far, I haven't been able to replicate a death deterring experience in a book. However, there is ample evidence that inadequate exercise can speed up the end of life as you know it. The following habit can contribute to a longer higher quality life.

Habit: Engage in some form of aerobic exercise for at least 30 minutes a day, six days a week, to stay firm, fit, and full of vitality.

Aerobic exercise is different from many of your daily activities, such as gardening or cleaning. Aerobic exercise consists of continuous, rhythmic activity that uses your large muscle groups and forces your heart and lungs to work harder than they do during your normal daily activities. When you strengthen your heart, it pumps blood more efficiently throughout your body. Your blood carries oxygen and nutrients to your brain and organs, and also ferries lactic acid, carbon dioxide, and other waste products away to be processed. The more efficiently your heart works, the better it is for the rest of your body.

Examples of aerobic exercise are brisk walking, jogging, running, stair-climbing, elliptical machine use, rowing, jumping rope, in-line skating, aerobic dancing, cycling, cross-country skiing, and swimming.

To achieve the benefits of aerobic exercise, it's not enough just to move continuously and rhythmically for 30 minutes (even though that's a good start for beginners). In order to gain the full benefits of aerobic exercise, you have to find your **target heart rate** and maintain it while you work out. A simple way to determine and maintain your target heart rate during exercise follows:

- Determine your maximum heart rate: Subtract your age from 220. Example: If you are 65 years-old, your maximum heart rate would be 155 beats per minute (220 - 65).

- Calculate your Target Heart Rate which is 65-80% of your maximum heart rate. Using the example above, your target heart rate would be 100 (65% of 155) to 124 (80% of 155) beats per minute.

- Take your pulse at your neck or wrist after you've been exercising for about 10 minutes. Count the beats for 10 seconds and multiply the result by 6 to figure out how many times your heart is beating every minute. If that number is between 100 and 124, maintain your level of exertion. If it's lower or higher, adjust your intensity to bring your heart rate up or down, as needed.

Important Note: The guidelines above are generally proven, acceptable measures of exercise exertion. However, as stated at the start of this book, it is essential to check with your health care professional before engaging in any exercise or nutritional program.

Studies show that people who participate in regular aerobic exercise live longer than those who don't exercise regularly. And, if you need some scientific evidence to be convinced, try this: The Copenhagen City Heart Study compared lifespans of joggers over their non-jogging counterparts. The 35-year study showed that jogging was associated with a lifespan increase of 6.2 years for men and 5.6 years for women. The joggers added those extra years by jogging 2 or 3 times a week to total 1 to 2.5 hours of jogging per week. In addition, over the 35-year study, there were 122 deaths among the joggers versus 10,158 deaths among the non-jogs. A final bit of encouraging news—the joggers reported being happier. Runners kick ass phalt!

- There are 10,080 minutes in every week. If you are 45 years old and you schedule 150 of those minutes in moderate exercise (25 minutes a day, 6 days a week) you **can gain 3.5 years of life**. The average American life expectancy is 78. An investment of 150 minutes a week over 33 years equals 4,290 hours in excerise (less than one half year).

- Your return, 3.5 additional years, is a 1 to 7 return! And, get this, strenuous exercise can approximately double the effect. For example, 75 minutes of jogging has roughly the effect of 150 minutes of brisk walking. So, instead, of gaining seven times the time spent, you'd be gaining 14 times.

(Source: Dr. I-Min Lee of Brigham and Women's Hosptial, Harvard professor and senior author of, "Leisure Time Physical Activity of Moderate to Vigorous Intensity and Mortality: A Large Pooled Cohort Analysis.")

Some additional benefits of regular aerobic exercise:

- Gets deep in your body, even into your DNA. Researchers have found that people who exercise have younger DNA by up to 9 years. That is an incredible benefit. So, exercising may do more than help prevent illness; it may make you younger.

- Increases your energy. Contrary to the belief that aerobic exercise can make you tired, it actually increases stamina and reduces fatigue over the long term.

- Helps manage high blood pressure and other chronic health conditions such as diabetes. If you've had a heart attack, aerobic exercise helps prevent subsequent attacks.

- Activates your immune system. I have not had the flu or a serious cold since I started my six-day-a-week aerobic exercise program 37 years ago.

- Reduces your risk of many serious health problems such as heart disease, obesity, type 2 diabetes, stroke, and certain types of cancer.

- Fights depression. It can reduce gloominess, decrease stress and tension, lessen anxiety, and promote relaxation.

- Contributes to your independence as you age. Aerobic exercise keeps your bones and muscles strong and contributes to balance and mobility.

Just in case you are not committed to adopting the daily exercise habit, you can add this benefit: it contributes to a more satisfying sex life.

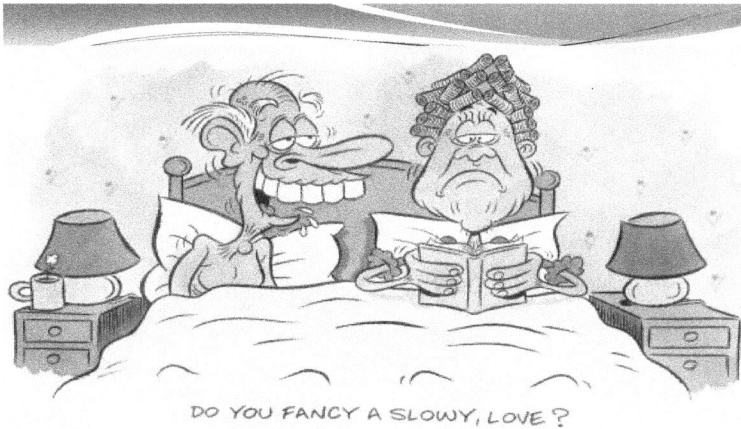

DO YOU FANCY A SLOWY, LOVE ?

In a Nutshell

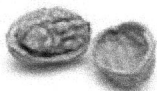

Make your minutes count! When you spend 150 minutes a week kickin' butt your payoff could be 3.5 extra years of energetic, disease-free, strong, and sexy life.

Chapter 14: Lift the Years Away

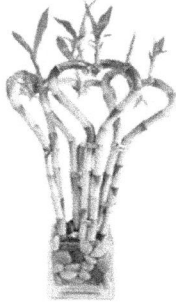

Take care of your body.
It is the only place you have to live in.
- Anon

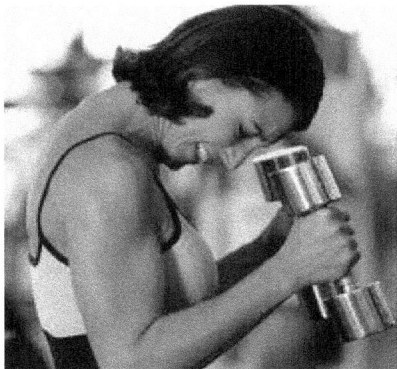

I discovered an exercise to help seniors build muscle strength in the arms and shoulders. It seems so easy, so I thought I'd pass it on to some of my friends and family. The manual suggested doing it three days a week.

Begin by standing on a comfortable surface, where you have plenty of room at each side. With a 5-pound potato sack in each hand, extend your arms straight out from your sides and hold them there as long as you can. Try to reach a full minute, then relax. Each day, you'll find that you can hold this position for just a bit longer.

After a couple of weeks, move up to a 10-pound potato sack. Then 50-lb potato sacks. Eventually try to get to where you can lift a 100-lb potato sack in each hand and hold your arms straight for more than a full minute. (I'm at this level).

After you feel confident at that level, put a potato in each of the sacks.

Habit: Strength training lifts my spirits, firms my body, and erases the years.

According to most exercise physiologists, we begin to lose about 1% of our muscle mass a year after puberty. Yikes! The best way to stop, prevent, **and reverse** bone and muscle loss is through strength training. Skyler Tanner, of Texas State University and author of ***Strength Training and its Effects on the Biomarkers of Aging,*** reports that strength training in the elderly reversed the aging process to the point that their genes got 10 years younger!

Strength training has a beneficial impact on six key biomarkers of aging: strength, muscle mass, blood pressure, bone density, cardiometabolic health (a strong, well-working heart that minimizes the risk of diabetes, heart disease or stroke), and metabolic syndrome (increased blood pressure, high sugar levels, increased belly fat and abnormal cholesterol levels). And, I'm confident that a 10 minute Google search will reveal that it can also improve your sex life! Combine the health benefits of strength training with the carnal benefits and you'll get a real bang for the buck (pun intended).

My personal strength training routine takes about 25 minutes (this includes the time it takes for a brief rest between sets) every other day. I alternate between upper body and lower body exercises. And, occasionally, I will do full-body exercises on one of the three days.

I also alternate my routines. One day, I'll do three sets of 15 reps each for each muscle group. The next time I lift, I'll increase the weight a little and do 8 reps going through the entire series before resting.

I follow a dumbbell routine that melts fat and builds muscle. It is available on www.popsugar.com (an excellent site for a wide variety of fitness information) and detailed below.

Important note: If you have not been engaged in a weight-training program, check with your doctor before starting and begin using 5 to 10 lb. weights.

Fil's Basic Weight Training Routine

I begin by spending about 10 minutes on the stationary bike, elliptical, or walking on the treadmill. The routine that follows takes about 20 minutes.

1. Lying Chest Fly. I like this particular pecs and chest lift because it also tones your lower abs.

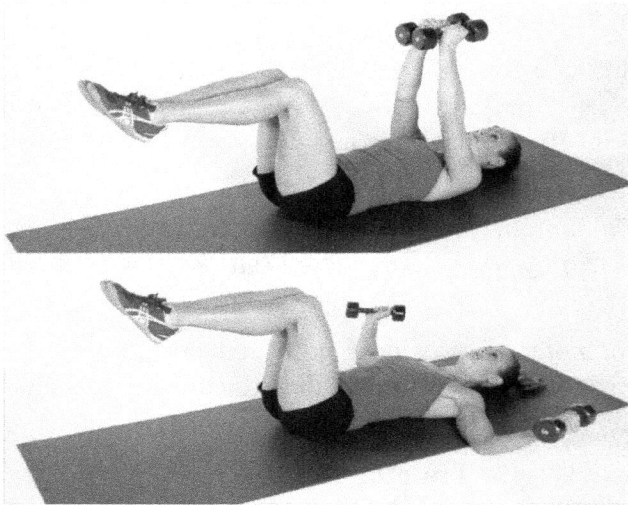

<u>1 rep</u>:

Lie on a mat with your back with hips and knees at 90 degree angles. Using your lower abs, press your lower back into the mat.

Raise your arms toward the ceiling, palms facing each other.

Keep your elbows slightly bent. Keep your midsection stable. Open your arms out to the side until your elbows are about 2 inches from the floor.

Raise your arms toward the ceiling; bring the weights together over your chest.

Do three sets of 10 reps.

2.   Lying Triceps Extension. Strengthens the backs of your arms.

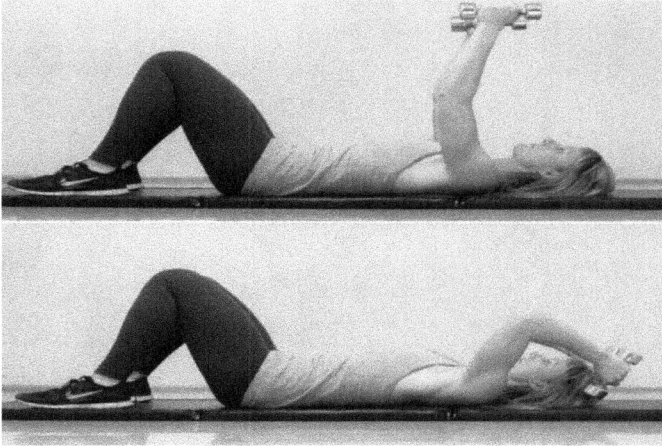

<u>1 rep:</u>

Lie on your back.

With a weight in each hand, raise your arms so they are above your chest. Make sure your elbows are straight but not locked.

Slowly lower both arms toward your head, bending your elbows to 90 degrees as the weights reach the mat. Aim to lower the weights so that they are on either side of your head. Keep elbows bent and pressing in toward your head.

Lift arms up to starting position.

Do three sets of 10 reps.

3. Squat, Curl & Press. Gets heart rate going. Works butt and legs.

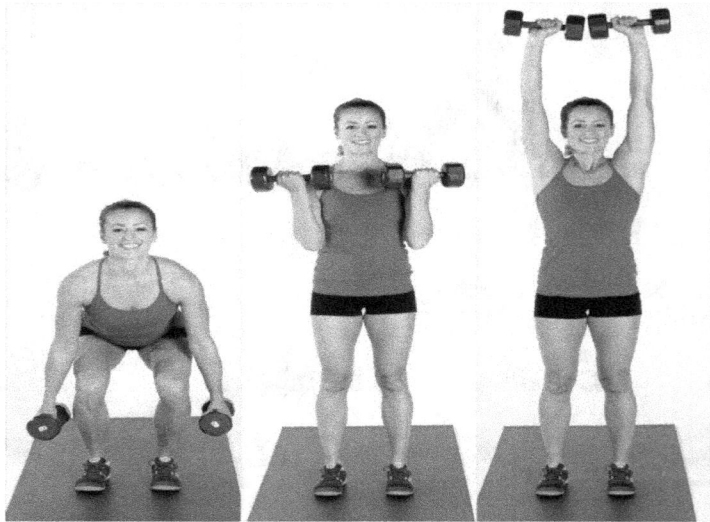

1 rep:

Stand with your feet directly under your hips. Hold a dumbbell in each hand. Sit back into a squat, keeping the weight in your heels. Bring your thighs parallel to the floor without letting your knees go beyond your toes.

Push through your heels to return to standing while bringing the weights to your shoulders, performing a bicep curl.

Stabilize your torso; move your arms upward, performing an overhead press with your palms facing out. Lower your arms back to your side.

Do three sets of 10 reps.

4. **Bent-over row**. Makes for shapely shoulders and a

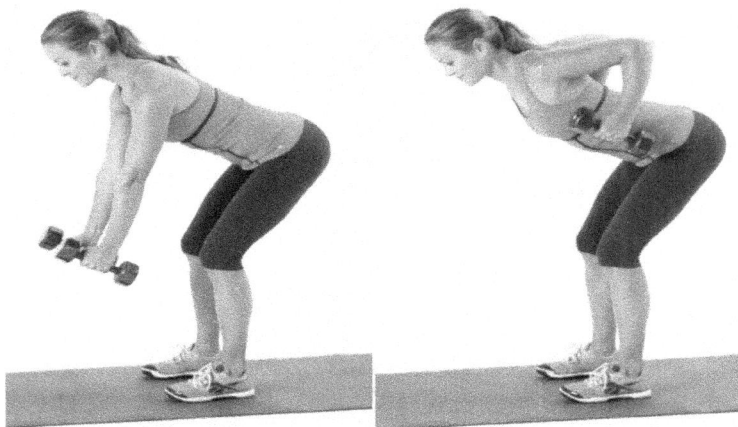

powerful back.

> *Note:* Use 10 to 15 lb. weights (if able to do so)

1 rep:

Lean forward and bend both knees. Keep your back flat.

Extend your arms so they are straight.

Lift the weights straight back to chest level, squeezing your shoulder blades together as you do. Keep your elbows in and pointed upward.

Slowly lower weights back to the starting position.

Do three sets of 10 reps.

5. Reverse Fly. Strengthens upper back.

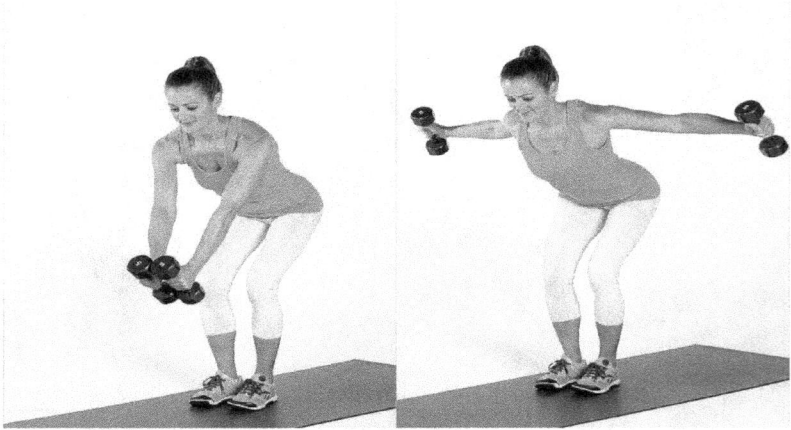

Note: Use 5 lb. weights

<u>1 rep</u>:

With a weight in each hand, stand with knees slightly bent. Keep back flat and bend forward at the hip joint.

Exhale and lift both arms to the side, maintaining a slight bend in the elbows and squeezing your shoulder blades together.

Then, with control, lower the weights back toward the ground.

Do three sets of 10 reps.

6. Lateral Raises. Strengthens shoulders, upper arms and upper back.

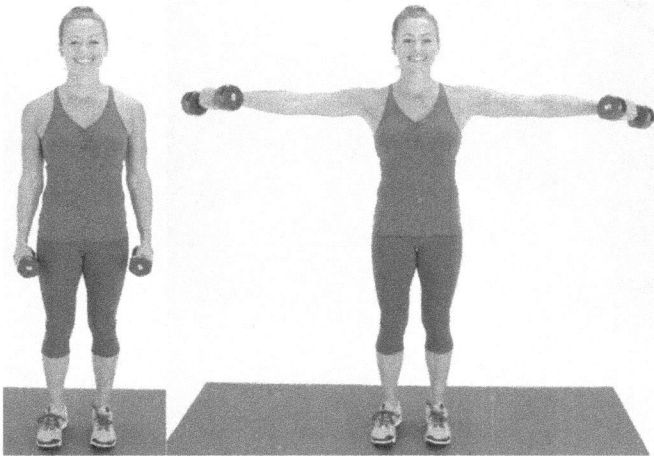

Note: Use 5 lb. weights

1 rep:

Stand with your feet hip's distance apart. Hold a weight in each hand so your palms face in toward the sides of your body.

Start with the right side first. With control, keep your arm straight (but don't lock the elbow). As you inhale, raise your right hand up toward the ceiling. You want your palm to be facing down and your arm to be parallel to the floor.

Then, as you exhale, slowly lower your hand back to your body. You should be able to see your hand in your peripheral vision. So your arm won't be directly out to the side, but slightly forward.

Do the same move with your left arm.

Then do both your right and left arms at the same time.

Continue these moves of right, left, together, right, left, together, for a total of 10 reps.

Do three sets of 10 reps.

To derive the maximum benefits from your strength training routine, I suggest you mix it up, changing:

- Your frequency

- Your routine

- Your weights—not only the pounds but the types, switching between free weights, machines, and resistance bands.

Just in case you forgot the "No Excuses" (chapter 1) and want to rationalize not engaging in strength training because you can't afford to join a gym or health club, fagedaboudit!

A set of free weights is relatively inexpensive and there are many objects around the average home that can be converted to an exercise bench. Even less expensive than free weights are resistance bands. An excellent site for ordering resistance bands at a good price AND for simple easy to follow instructions for using them is www.workoutz.com.

There are many web sites that illustrate strength training. Two of them that provide easy-to-follow guides are:

http://www.sparkpeople.com/resource/fitness.asp
http://www.exercise.about.com

Banish the archaic belief that strength training is about muscleheads and bodybuilders sweating it out at Gold's Gym. It benefits people of all ages and physical conditions including those with age-related health issues such as arthritis and heart conditions.

In a Nutshell

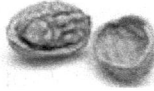

Strength training can benefit your heart, improve your balance, strengthen your bones, help you lose weight AND make you years younger. It definitely makes you look and feel better! There are not many things more attractive than a fit, well-toned body.

Twenty-five minutes of strength training every other day can prevent, retard, and even reverse bone and muscle loss. It is a cheap and easy way to look and feel fit.

Chapter 15: Mind Your Middle

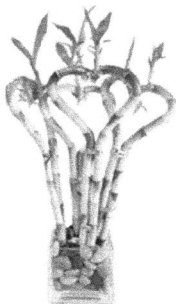

All those guys with 6-pack abs,
and I'm the one with a keg.
- Homer Simpson

Many people think that core training is simply another name for abdominal exercises aimed at getting a six-pack. This is incorrect.

Core training is about training your body's foundation—the muscles that support good posture and efficient movement. Core training does not focus on a single muscle, but rather focuses on improving how the muscles at the center of your body work together to provide you with stability, balance, and control over your movement.

A weak core makes you susceptible to lower back pain, poor posture, and a whole host of muscle injuries.

Strong core muscles help prevent such pain and injury. In addition, a strong core provides the following benefits:

- Better posture

- Good carriage

- Improved control over body movements

- Faster rehabilitation from injuries

- Increased protection and "bracing" for your back

- A more stable center of gravity

- A hot bod!

My "core habit" is: I enjoy my core training. It whittles my middle, keeps me stable and balanced, and keeps back pain at bay.

I do core exercises every other day for 20 min. My personal routine is listed below. I do two sets of 40 reps each. However, I want to be quick to point out that I started at two sets of 10 reps each.

1. Warm up with a full body stretch.

Lie flat on your back with your legs extended and your arms stretched overhead. Relax your abs. Stretch through the center of your body by stretching your toes and fingertips towards opposite sides of the room.

Breathe deeply and hold for 10-30 seconds.

An important note: Stretch to the point of "mild discomfort," not to the point of pain. Never bounce. Don't allow your lower back to arch off of the floor or mat.

Do three sets of 10 reps each.

2. Pelvic tilt.

Lie on your back, knees bent, feet flat on the floor, and hands either by your sides or supporting your head.

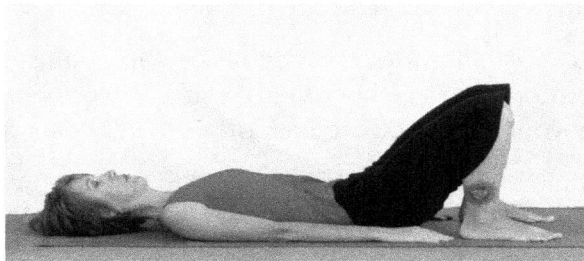

Firmly tighten your bottom, forcing your lower back flat against the floor.

Relax and repeat

Do three sets of 10 reps each.

3. Crunches.

Lie down on your back with your knees bent. Place your hands on your head right behind your ears.

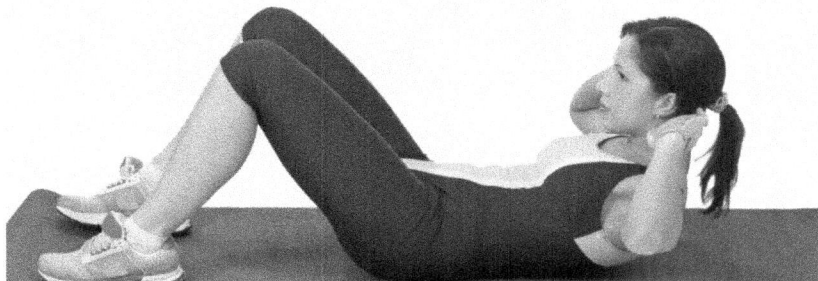

While breathing out, contract your abdominal muscles to lift your head, neck, and shoulders off the floor and curl forward no more than 45 degrees.

Hold for a moment before returning to the starting position, then repeat.

Do three sets of 10 reps each.

4. Reverse Crunch.

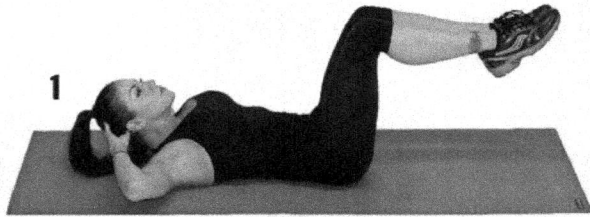

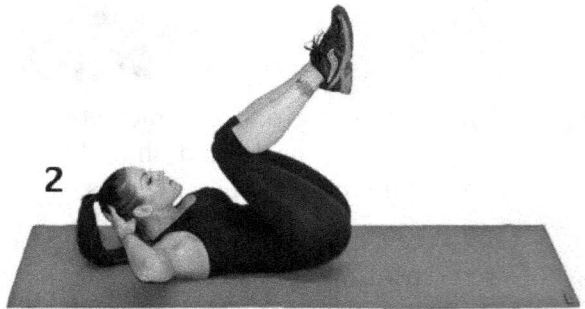

1. Lie on your back and extend your arms out to the side and raise your knees and feet so they create a 90-degree angle.

2. Contract your abdominals and exhale as you lift your hips off the floor with control; moving your knees toward your head. Keep your knees at a right angle. Inhale and slowly lower.

Do three sets of 10 reps each.

5. Oblique crunches.

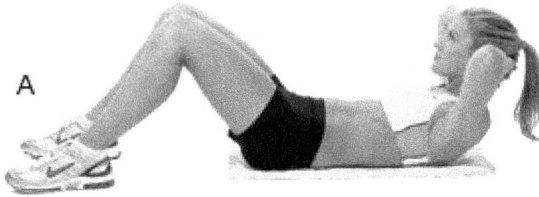

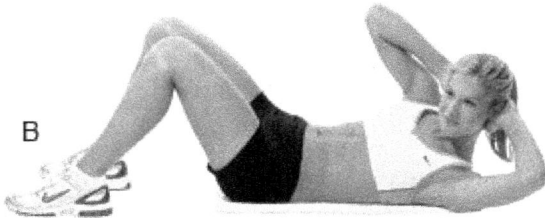

Lie on your back with your legs bent, your feet flat on the floor, and your hands behind your head.

Lift your right shoulder off the floor and bring your right elbow across your body toward your left knee.

Repeat on the opposite side, moving your left elbow toward your right knee.

Do three sets of 10 reps each.

Important note: Keep your head in a neutral position and relax your neck to ensure that the contraction is in your abdomen area only.

6. Low back strengthener.

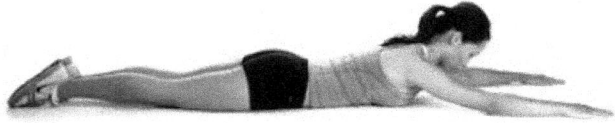

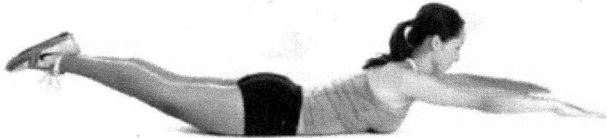

Lie on your stomach with your arms straight over your head, your chin resting on the floor between your arms.

Keeping your arms and legs straight, simultaneously lift your feet and your hands as high off the floor as you can (aim for at least three inches off the floor).

Hold that position (sort of a Superman flying position) for 10 seconds if possible, and then relax your arms and legs back on to the floor.

If this exercise is too difficult to start, try lifting just your legs or arms off the floor separately, or even just one limb at a time.

Do three sets of 10 reps each.

7. Modified push-ups.

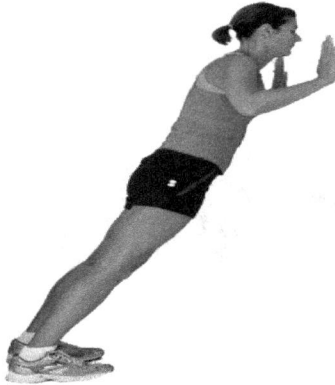

Stand about 3 feet in front of a wall with your hands outstretched and touching the wall. Lean your body towards the wall

Push your body back, with your hands until you are once again in a standing position.

Repeat 10 times keeping an even rhythm up and back.

Do three sets of 10 reps each.

8. Plank.

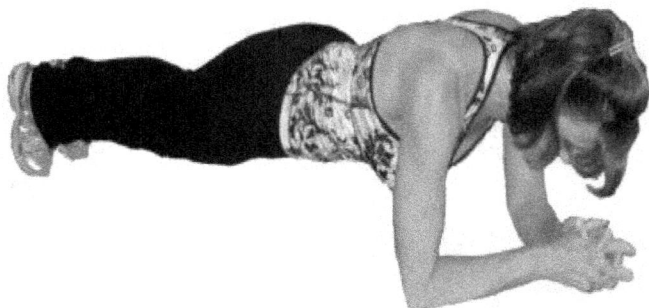

Lie face down. Lift your body, resting your weight on your forearms and toes.

Hold or 'hover' (30-90 sec) keeping your body in a straight line from your shoulders to your ankles.

Return to starting position.

Do three sets of 10 reps each.

Tips: Keep your bum in line with the rest of your body. If possible, do the plank exercise in front of a mirror to make sure your body says "plank" - not "spank."

Variation: Do the plank on a stability ball. Work up to 60 seconds...or better yet, 90!

There are a variety of ways to get instructional information about core exercises. A personal trainer is the ideal. However, you can find a variety of easy to follow core exercises by googling how to do "core exercises." Or go to http://www.mayoclinic.com/health/core-strength/SM00047 for an illustrated series. Another on-line resource is http://www.shapefit.com/abs/ab-workouts.html.

In a Nutshell

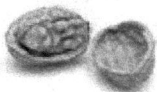

Twenty minutes of core training every other day is an essential anti-aging exercise because your core muscles support good posture, stability, balance, and control over your movement.

Chapter 16: Stay Limber, Lithe, and Lively

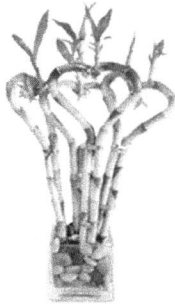

If your spine is inflexibly stiff at 30, you are old;
if it is completely flexible at 60, you are young.
- Joseph H. Pilates

As you age, your muscles tighten and the range of motion in the joints can be constricted. This can put a damper on active lifestyles and even hinder day-to-day, normal motions.

My personal stretch habit is: Ten minutes of daily stretching contributes to my life-long independence; the ability to take care of myself, live where I want to, and the way I want to as long as I live.

The beauty of stretching is that you don't need special equipment, a gym membership, or expensive shoes. You don't have to pack extra items when you travel and you can do it just about anywhere.

My favorite places to stretch: The backyard, on the beach, in my office and—when I'm living dangerously—when I'm waiting in line.

I love to dance. A quote from Scott Adams, the Dilbert cartoonist: *Dance like it hurts...love like you need money...work when people are watching*, speaks to the importance of stretching. So many people who want to be lively and shake a tail feather are limited by tight muscles and reduced range of motion. They "Dance like it hurts."

A good, easy to follow, illustrated stretching routine, "10 Stretches You can do Anywhere" appears below and is available   at http://www.sparkpeople.com/resource/articles_print.asp?id=12 64.

Hold each stretch listed for 15-30 seconds, repeating two or three times, depending on how you feel. For detailed instructions and larger photos, click on the name of each stretch. Please note that while some of these stretches depict various body positions, you can perform the upper body stretches while sitting in a chair.

Neck Stretch

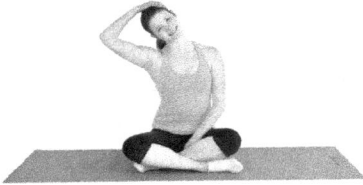

Sit or stand with shoulders relaxed, back straight. Bring your left ear down toward your left shoulder and hold. Roll your head down toward the ground and bring your chin to your chest. Hold and finally, roll your head to the right and bring your right ear to your right shoulder. Inhale and exhale in a slow and controlled manner.

Chest Stretch

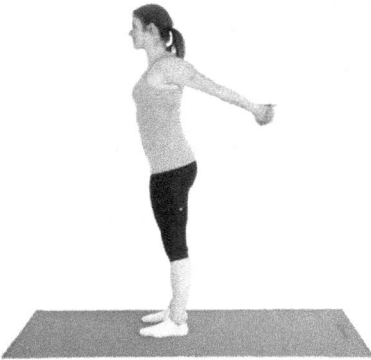

Stand tall or sit upright (not pictured). Interlace your fingers behind your back and straighten your arms. With arms straight, lift your arms up behind you while keeping your back straight and your shoulders down. Keep your shoulders relaxed away from your ears.

Standing Triceps Stretch

Stand tall or sit upright (not pictured). Place your left elbow in your right hand. Reach your left arm overhead, placing your left palm on the center of your back and supporting your elbow in your right hand. Reach your fingertips down your spine. Keep your shoulders relaxed away from your ears. Repeat with your opposite arm.

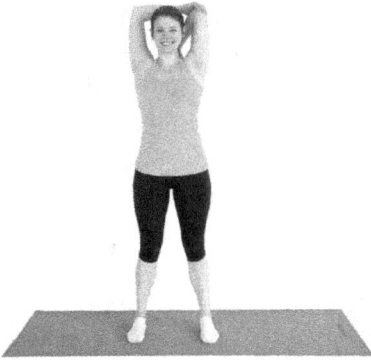

Shoulder Stretch

Stand tall or sit upright (not pictured). Bring your left arm across your chest, holding it below the elbow with your opposite hand. Keep your shoulders relaxed away from your ears. Breathe deeply and hold. Repeat on the opposite side.

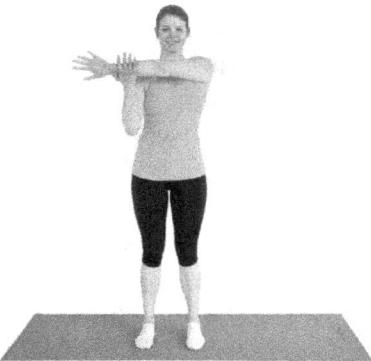

Wrist and Biceps Stretch

Stand tall or sit upright (not pictured). Extend your left arm in front of you with palm facing outward and fingertips pointing downward. Use your right hand to apply light pressure to your left hand, as if pulling your fingertips toward your elbow. Keep shoulders relaxed away from your ears. Breathe deeply and hold. Repeat on opposite side.

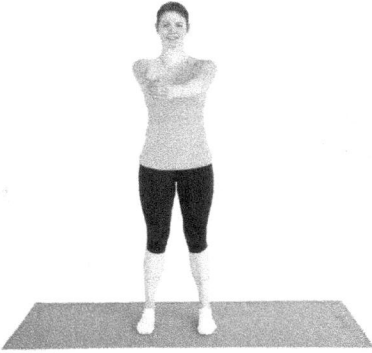

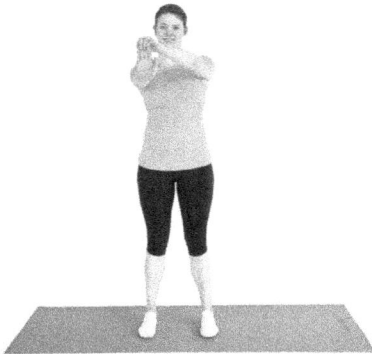

Wrist and Forearm Stretch

Stand tall or sit upright (not pictured). Extend your left arm in front of you, palm facing outward and fingertips pointing upward. Use your right hand to apply light pressure to the hand, as if pulling your fingertips toward your shoulder. Keep shoulders relaxed away from your ears. Breathe deeply and hold. Repeat on opposite side.

121

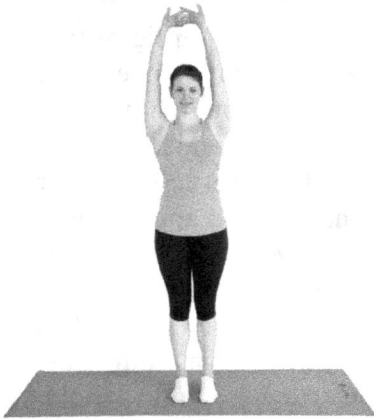

Torso Stretch

Clasp your hands together and slowly raise them above your head toward the ceiling. Reach as high as you can while inhaling deeply. Hold for 20-30 seconds. Bring your hands down slowly while letting out your breath.

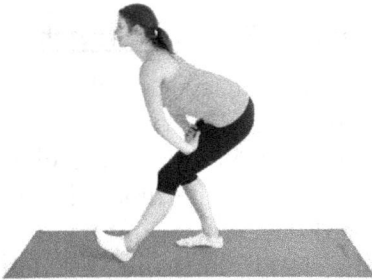

Hamstring Stretch

Stand tall with your back straight, abs engaged, shoulders down, and feet hip-width apart. Bring your left leg forward, heel down, toes up and leg straight. Keep your back straight and abs engaged as you bend your right knee as if sitting back, while supporting yourself with both hands on your thighs. Repeat on the opposite side.

Quad Stretch

Stand tall, holding onto a chair or wall for balance if necessary (not pictured). Keep your feet hip-width apart, your back straight and your feet parallel. Reach back and grab your left foot with your left hand, keeping your thighs lined up next to each other and your left leg in line with your hip (not pulled back behind you). Repeat on the opposite side.

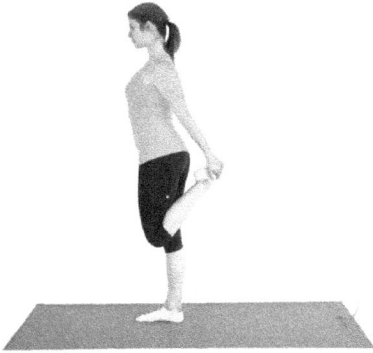

Inner Thigh Stretch

Stand tall with your back straight, feet wider than the hips, toes turned out, abs engaged and arms at your sides. Slowly bend your knees, squatting straight down, hands supported on your thighs, until you feel a stretch through your inner thighs.

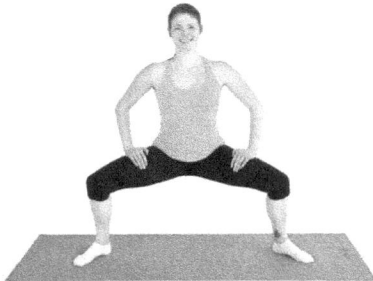

Ten minutes of stretching every day pays off big-time with:

- Better balance/flexibility.

- Reduced muscle tension.

- Increased range of movement in the joints.

- Enhanced muscular coordination.

- Increased circulation of the blood to various parts of the body.

- Increased energy levels (the result of increased circulation).

In a Nutshell

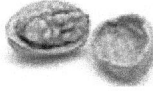

Ten minutes of stretching every day can keep you lithe and lively all of your life. Depending where you elect to stretch, you can also brighten another person's day!

Chapter 17: Jump for Life or Skip it!

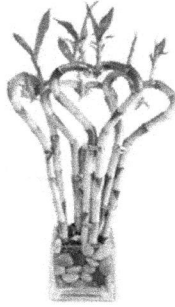

Jack be nimble. Jack be quick.
Jack jump over the candlestick.
- Mother Goose

If you are someone who instinctively moves to the rhythm, it is easy to form a habit similar to my own:

Habit: I jump for life and skip for joy.

And, because I exercise with my iPod, the music moves me to jump and/or skip at least 3 times a week.

Jumping rope and skipping are two of the highest calorie burning exercises! I love them both for several reasons, not the least of which is I don't need any expensive equipment or a gym membership.

Let's start with jumping rope. Did you know that:

• Jumping rope for 10 minutes is the cardiovascular equivalent of jogging for half an hour **and** 10 minutes of jumping rope burns the same amount of calories as 30 minutes of jogging!

• The repetitive motions you experience while jumping rope help you feel more relaxed and focused.

• Jumping activates the lymphatic system. The lymphatic system is like your body's sewer system. It removes all sorts of waste and toxins from your blood and moves them out to be eliminated. However, unlike your circulatory system, the lymphatic system doesn't have a pump. It relies on the expansion and contraction of your muscles to move and eliminate waste and toxins.

• A healthy, circulating lymphatic system is essential for healthy, beautiful skin. And it just so happens that the up and down motion of jumping rope is one of the best exercises for moving the lymph system. Jumping on a trampoline provides the same benefit.

• Beyond long-term fitness benefits, jumping rope can also relieve stress. This is because jumping rope can produce an endorphin buzz. Endorphins are biochemical substances produced by the pituitary gland and hypothalamus during strenuous exercise. Endorphins are the body's natural opiates. They can reduce pain and bring about a feeling of euphoria and well-being. When you are at the end of your rope, jump it!

Although jumping rope is similar to running, it doesn't cause the same strain on your muscular-skeletal system when done correctly. You can find an excellent video tutorial, "Learn How to Jump Rope," on-line at www.BuiltLean.com. To their top-notch advice, I would add:

- **Start without a rope.** Use an imaginary rope to start. This will keep you from jumping too high. Even if you begin with a rope, adjust the length so that you hold it about hip high. Use your wrists to turn the rope. When you rely on your arms or shoulders to turn the rope, it makes it unnecessarily difficult.

- **Aim for about half a minute or one minute to start.** You can gradually build up to a longer period of time.

- **Keep your head up and back straight, knees slightly bent, and jump on the balls of your feet.** Don't let your heels touch the ground.

- **Jump to the Beat**

Do you remember?

Teddy Bear, Teddy Bear, turn around

Teddy Bear, Teddy Bear, touch the ground

Teddy Bear, Teddy Bear, tie your shoe

Teddy Bear, Teddy Bear, please skiddo!

And

Johnny gave me apples,

Johnny gave me pears.

Johnny gave me fifty cents

To kiss him on the stairs.

I gave him back his apples,

I gave him back his pears.

I gave him back his fifty cents

And kicked him down the stairs.

Jumping to the beat makes it easier and fun!

Just a few of the benefits of jumping rope:

- Increased bone and muscle strength.
- Greater bone density.
- Stronger core.
- Better balance and posture.
- Improved coordination and reflexes.

Important Note: It is essential to consult with your physician before starting to jump rope or skip. Once you have your doctor's approval, remember to start out slow to gain the maximum benefits and avoid injury.

Skipping is a terrific way to break the monotony of working out on an elliptical machine or stationary bike. And, I can tell you from personal experience it breaks the monotony of everyday life for others as well. I was spotted by a business associate while skipping on the beach in Cape May, New Jersey more than a decade ago. Whenever we meet, he asks me if I am still skipping.

Just in case you think skipping is childish—it is! When I skip, I can't help but smile and reminisce about a time when life was freer, simpler, and full of promise. And, if the lore of childhood memories doesn't appeal to you, consider these benefits:

- **Physical Benefits:** You can burn up to 900 calories per hour. Skipping improves your cardiovascular system, strengthens your lower body muscles, improves coordination, flexibility, and balance.

- **Brain Functioning:** Because skipping requires a constant level of coordination and cross lateral processing, it can significantly enhance brain functioning.

- **Enhanced bone density:** Skipping for as little as 2-5 minutes per day can significantly boost bone density levels that could reduce or eliminate the onset of osteoporosis.

If you want to form an exercise habit that is a little different, fun, free and allows you to glide past some of the adverse effects of aging, skip!

In a Nutshell

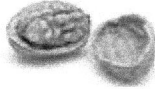

Two inexpensive, useful exercises that result in cardiovascular fitness, weight control, and brain health are jumping rope and skipping.

When you use proper form, jumping rope can be easier on your muscular/skeletal system than jogging.

It is important to get your physician's approval before embarking on either one of these exercises, just as it is with all exercise programs.

Both jumping rope and skipping are more fun when done to music or "the beat" of a rhyme.

Chapter 18: Dance like Nobody's Watching

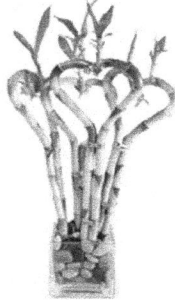

The one thing that can solve most of our problems is dancing.
- James Brown

Follow the advice in this chapter to bring joy to yourself and others while keeping your brain and your body healthy.

Let's start with a quick quiz. Albert Einstein College of Medicine conducted a 21-year study of people 75 years and older. The purpose of the study was to see if any physical or cognitive recreational activities influenced mental acuity. The activities they studied included reading books, writing for pleasure, doing crossword puzzles, playing cards, playing musical instruments, playing tennis or golf, swimming, bicycling, dancing, walking for exercise, and doing housework.

Can you correctly match the reduced risk of dementia to each of the activities listed below?

Instructions: Match each activity on the left to the correct degree to which it reduces the risk of dementia on the right.

Activity	Reduced risk of dementia
Reading	0%
Dancing frequently	35%
Doing crossword puzzles at least 4 days a week	0%
Playing golf	47%
Bicycling and swimming	76%

See answers on page 135.

I love to dance! And, now that I have passed the three-quarters of a century mark, I have overcome the four main barriers that prevent people from enjoying the longevity benefits of dance. My dance habits purposely eliminate those barriers:

    1.   **Habit: Age and self-consciousness do not render me incapable of memorizing more than two dance steps in a row.** Others are too busy stumbling over their own dorkiness than to be watching mine.

2.   Habit: I give people at the mall a lift when I boogie at Bloomies.

3.   Habit: I accept that sitting on my ass watching *Dancing with the Stars* and *So You Think you Can Dance* does not constitute a weight loss program. I dance with them!

4.   Habit: I dance to feel free, happy and independent!

Liberated, now I can enjoy the benefits of dance, some of which may surprise you. Frequent dancing can:

- **Relieve Stress**

Dancing truly does lift your spirits! A controlled study cited in the Journal of Applied Gerontology reported that partner dance and musical accompaniment can reduce stress.

- **Reduce the risk of dementia**

Why does dancing produce the greatest reduction in the risk of dementia? According to Harvard Medical School Psychiatrist Dr. Joseph Coyle: "The cerebral cortex and hippocampus, which are critical to dance, are remarkably plastic, and they rewire themselves based upon their use." Our brain constantly rewires its neural pathways, as needed. If it doesn't need to, then it won't. Dancing can put that process to work. If for no other reason, dance to deter dementia.

Answers to quiz on top of page 133.

Activity	Reduced risk of dementia
Dancing frequently	**76%**
Doing crossword puzzles at least 4 days a week	47%
Reading	35%
Bicycling and swimming	0%
Playing golf	0%

- **Give you Greater Vitality**

Feeling blah and listless? No get-up-and-go? Dancing might help. Research published in the ***Scholarly Publishing and Academic Resources Coalition*** reported that a weekly dance program could improve physical performance and **increase energy levels** of adults.

- **Change the way you think**

Dr Peter Lovatt is head of the Dance Psychology Lab at the University of Hertfordshire. Dr. Lovatt studied people in the lab dancing and then doing problem solving. What he discovered was that when people did improvised dancing, it helped them with divergent thinking—a thought process or method used to generate creative ideas by exploring a number of different possible solutions. Dr. Lovatt also discovered that when people engaged in structured dance, they were better able to do convergent thinking—trying to find the single right answer to a problem.

Another fascinating aspect of Dr. Lovatt's dance research relates to people with Parkinson's disease, which - as it develops - can lead to a disruption of divergent thinking. When Dr. Lovatt used improvised dance with a group of Parkinson's patients, they gained an improvement in their divergent thinking skills.

- **Contribute to independence**

Dance builds flexibility and grace. Flexible people are less likely to experience falls. I now know why, when I visit my primary care physician, I'm asked if I've fallen recently. That is because three out of ten people over 65 suffer falls. One bad fall and your ability to live independently is threatened.

- **Make friends**

A dance class is ideal for making new friends. When we dance, we are honest, free and expressive. And, it is fun. Positive relationships rank high on the contributors to longevity; they are right up there with healthy nutrition and exercise. In fact, lack of positive social relationships can have as negative an impact on life expectancy as smoking!

- **Make Whoopie**

Dancing with another is a form of intimate communication. It requires that you respond to, support, and be engaged with each other, all of which could lead to something beautiful!

Where can you dance? Anywhere your heart desires. We don't do enough street dancing in this country. You can find classes at a fitness center, the gym, or a dance studio. Or, you can do basic aerobic dance anywhere. The only equipment you will need is some rockin' music. A great resource for basic aerobic dance moves, is http://www.livestrong.com/article/108576-list-aerobic-steps/#ixzz2GLqKSBlU.

Every day brings a chance for you to draw in a breath,
kick off your shoes, and dance.
- Oprah Winfrey

In a Nutshell

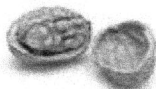

One of the greatest benefits of dancing is that it has been proven to reduce the risk of dementia. It has a greater impact than a vast majority of other mental and physical activities.

You don't need to be good at dance to derive all of the benefits.

When you dance frequently, you can relieve stress, increase vitality, change the way you think, stay independent, make friends, and improve your sex life.

Section IV:
The Joy Factor

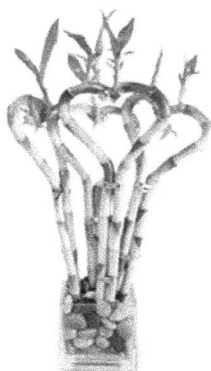

How to capture the joy of a love affair with life.

Chapter 19: Lighten Up!

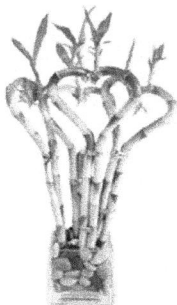

Choose to be optimistic, it feels better.
- Dalai Lama

A Johns Hopkins 25-year study on heart disease revealed a link between a positive outlook on life and a measurable reduction in cardiac events, including heart attacks. In fact, positive well-being was associated with a one-third reduction in coronary events.

Being optimistic, like many other aspects of our physical and psychological makeup, may be in our genes. However, genetics does not play as significant a role in longevity as most people think. According to the Centers for Disease Control, lifestyle has more than twice the impact of hereditary influences. Here is their assessment of the major factors:

- 20% Genetics
- 20% Environment

- 10% Health Care
- 50% Lifestyle

So, even though a positive personality may be part of the temperament you are born with, you can adopt habits that can change that. You can "choose to be optimistic" as advocated by the Dalai Lama.

Choosing optimism is like deciding to eat clean or to exercise regularly: all three are lifestyle choices.

My habit: I greet each day with joy in my heart. I am open to the good in people, and events, and I do good.

Just a few of the ways I choose to be upbeat:

Sing! There have been some remarkable new discoveries about the brain and singing. In the book, *This is Your Brain on Music* by Daniel Levitin, professor of neurochemistry at McGill University, cites a number of studies that show that singing elevates the levels of neurotransmitters associated with pleasure and well-being. People's levels of oxytocin, the transmitter associated with pleasure, love and bonding, were measured before and after voice lessons. Oxytocin levels increased significantly after lessons for both amateur and professional singers.

Our brains reward us with good feelings after singing and with good reason. Our brains developed along with song and music as a survival mechanism. Our ancient ancestors used songs and dance to build loyalty, transmit vital information and ward off enemies. You sang well; you survived!

My habit: It doesn't matter whether I sing well or not. I break into spontaneous song. It's good for my brain and my spirit.

Another benefit of song: It can strengthen your immune system. Researchers at the University of Frankfurt in Germany tested the blood of people who sang in a professional choir before and after a 60-minute rehearsal of Mozart's Requiem. Their findings, published in the **US *Journal of Behavioral Medicine,*** reported concentrations of immunoglobin A (proteins in the immune system which function as antibodies) and hydrocortisone (an anti-stress hormone) increased significantly during the rehearsal. A week later, they asked members of the choir to listen to a recording of the Requiem without singing. The result: The composition of their blood did not change significantly; it still showed signs of a strengthened immune system. Just listening to song has health benefits.

Sing a new song. Resist the old tapes that play in your head. You know the ones that are entitled *I'm getting old, I really screwed up, I can't stick with an exercise routine, I don't have any energy, blah, blah, blah.* Replace them with self-affirming tunes *I am ever-young, My energy is boundless, I am a regular, disciplined, happy exerciser...*

Smile! Contrary to popular belief, we don't smile because we are happy. Instead, we are happy because we smile. Scientist and happiness expert, Robert Azjonc, conducted a series of studies in which he proved that smiling causes physiological changes that create the sensation of happiness and that frowning can bring about changes that make you feel sad. According to Zajonc, when you smile it causes changes in your brain and blood that make you feel happy. Actions trigger feelings, so the simple feel good action of smiling can make you feel happier.

Smile even more. Because smiling not only makes you feel good, it causes positive feelings in others. When others see you smiling, they are more likely to perceive you as being a pleasant person and will treat you accordingly. For example, studies show that smiling servers in restaurants get the largest tips. Smiling feels good and it also reminds us to stay positive and communicate our affirmative feelings to others, encouraging them to feel happy as well.

Oh hell! Even Laugh. Laughter prolongs your life. It increases blood circulation by more than 20% and prevents hardening of the arteries, according to University of Maryland School of Medicine researchers. They recommend a minimum of 15 minutes of laughter daily.

Try mental Feng Shui. An e-mail called Mental Feng Shui circulated a few years ago with excellent advice for life. Number 20 states *as soon as you realize you've made a mistake do something to correct it.* (Goggle Mental Feng Shui to read the entire list.) Mistakes or missteps are actions that result in unintended outcomes. Typically, those consequences cause problems or pain for others. Don't waste energy defending your actions! Most people don't care what motivated you to do what you did, nor are they interested in your intentions vs. your behavior. Defensiveness saps positive energy that would be better invested in correcting your mistake. Next time you misstep, acknowledge it, express regret, and ask forgiveness. Your inner light will show through, and you'll have more energy to do something to correct your error.

Call out the positive in others. Consciously look for and acknowledge a positive attribute in each and every person you encounter, including family, friends, and loved ones. Make it personal and specific. We rarely take the time to give the kind of compliment that highlights another's positive attributes. Things like: *I appreciate having you as a neighbor; you are always willing to lend a helping hand,* or *you brighten my day with your funny stories.* Test the concept. Begin today and keep it up for 21 days.

In a Nutshell

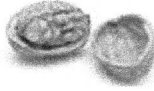

Give voice to the music in your head. Song was one of the earliest brain builders. Sing to keep your brain sharp and your immune system strong.

Record some new tapes to replace the old ones (I can't, I'm not good/smart/pretty/handsome/young enough) with updated positive messages.

Smile. You will feel better and so will others.

Laugh for 15 minutes a day, even if it makes soda come out of your nose!

Apologize instead of defending your missteps.

Look for and acknowledge the positives in others.

Chapter 20: Sex - Get it On and Get it Off

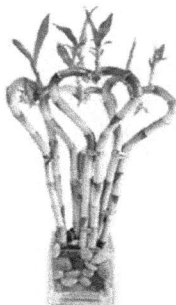

If the authorities on aging warn you of the dangers of having sex, heed their advice and don't have sex with the authorities!

When one of the geriatric doctors I worked with writing this book advised me to include "senior sex," I hesitated for at least 30 seconds. *"Why not?"* I thought. The sex act got us here. Then on the very same day, and this is why I believe that the cosmos acts in our favor if we only pay attention, I stumbled upon two articles reporting that sexual satisfaction in older adults can add life to your years! It got us here AND can keep us here!

In the first article from ***Health Day News,*** researchers at the Stein Institute for Research on Aging at the University of California, San Diego School of Medicine, reported the results of a study of 1,200 women aged 60-89. They found that sexual satisfaction was **not** associated with age. In fact, satisfaction with overall sex life was reported by 67% of those aged 60-69; 60% of those aged 70-79; and 61% of those aged 80-89! And here is the bonus according to the study, "although the levels of sexual activity and functioning did vary significantly, depending on the women's age, their perceived quality of life, successful aging and sexual satisfaction remained positive."

You probably don't need any more encouragement to get it on. But, here are a few more bennies, according to Dr. Michael Roizen and Dr. Mehmet Oz:

- Women who enjoy sex live longer lives than women who do not.

- Sex can make women feel two to eight years younger.

- General pain can be decreased through orgasms.

The second article posted on RealAge.com reported that men with a high frequency of orgasms have a 50 percent reduction in mortality risk.

My four habits for a longer, healthier, happier sex life as I age:

- **Habit: I Love my body**. I exercise, maintain a healthy weight and blood pressure, and am not at all concerned that my body is not perfect. It is the body I have and it doesn't need to be perfect to deliver the perfect experience.

- **Habit: I'm mercilessly open and honest.** I talk to my partner about my needs and desires. AND, I don't hesitate to take things into my own hands.

- **Habit: I talk to my Doc.** I am willing to discuss any health related barriers to good sex with my primary care physician.

- **Habit: I abandon discretion**. I prefer to be dyslexic: Sex on the spot is just as exciting at 74 as it is at 47!

Having more sex may increase how long you live. Even if it doesn't add years to your life, sex can sure add life to your years. Just a few of the benefits:

- According to scientists at Princeton University, having regular sex may help us grow new brain cells. Good news considering that at age 35, we start to lose brain cells at the rate of about 7,000 a day. It seems that the more sex you have, the more cells you can grow. Animal studies, published in the journal *PLoS ONE*, suggest that sex stimulates the growth of brain cells in the hippocampus, the part of the brain responsible for memory and learning. Also, there is some evidence that older people who are sexually active are less likely to have dementia.

- Sex has also been reported to boost brain cells due to a surge in sex hormones, particularly testosterone, which can help improve concentration and reaction times.

- The endorphins released during sex can help lessen depression and clear the mind.

In a Nutshell

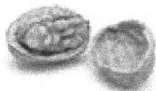

Sex is kicking death in the ass while singing.
-Charles Bukowski

Chapter 21: Unload!

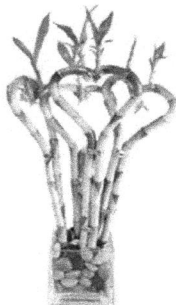

One of the secrets of a long and fruitful life is to forgive
everybody everything every night before you go to bed.
- Bernard Baruch

One of my goals way back when I first adopted Maltz's Cybernetics was I have a warm, loving, mutually rewarding relationship with my son. Jay was struggling with undiagnosed bipolar disorder and substance abuse. I was feeling angry, resentful, and betrayed. Today Jay is a successful, caring, responsible son, husband, father, and grandfather. At the time, I was relatively young and had no idea there was a link between forgiveness and longevity. More recently, researchers at the University of Tennessee conducted studies on the effect of having a forgiving personality and a longer life. Their findings suggest that harboring feelings of betrayal may be linked to stroke, kidney or heart failure, or even death.

The best way to describe my relationship with Jay is by recounting the classic fable of two monks:

Two monks, on a journey, came to a stream. The current was strong and the water deep. At the time, a young woman was also at the water's edge, wary of crossing. All needed to get to the other side. One of the monks picked her up, carried her across and placed her gently on the other side.

The monks continued in silence for a number of miles. Finally, one monk spoke. "You know it is against the rules to have contact with a woman. How could you do that?" To which the first replied, "I put that woman down miles ago, it is you who has been carrying her this whole time."

I was carrying disappointment, dashed hopes and aspirations. **And,** was also attempting to control Jay in order to get what I wanted. Once I was able to unload, to put down my hurt, worries, and concerns about my son, and my personal regrets about what I had done or not done to contribute to his addiction, I began to see glimmers of that *warm, loving, mutually rewarding* relationship.

This is a good point at which to refer to one of my earlier proclamations. Although I was able to unload and "walk down a different street" by adopting the habits of forgiveness, it took more than 21 days for my ideal state to manifest, it took years. The resultant joy came from the following habits:

Habit: Abandon the right to resentment, negative judgment, and blaming toward the one who has hurt you and give the gift of forgiveness.

It would be a bold-faced lie to claim that I wasn't pissed at my son. And, if he hadn't emerged from my own womb, I might be serving a life sentence right now. What helped me unload my anger was to remind myself that forgiveness was not a pardon or an excuse for Jay's behavior nor did it condone it. Instead, I adopted the view that it was the circumstances in which Jay found himself and not his underlying personality or his desire to hurt me that lead to his actions. So, in my mind and my prayers, I gave him the gift of forgiveness. When his progress didn't go as I had hoped, or new problems arose, I kept reminding myself that even though he was hurting he had to find his own way and that my forgiveness might in someway make the path less arduous.

Habit: Put down the guilt you lay on yourself and give yourself the gift of forgiveness.

Many sleepless nights gave me ample time to figure out that blaming myself allowed me to wallow in self-pity, fear and regret. Letting go of the guilt did not come effortlessly. What I did and didn't do in raising my son kept haunting me. I needed a permission slip to stop blaming myself. The release finally came when I started to think about my errors in terms of the causes. Were my mistakes due to my circumstances? Were they due to my moral shortcomings? Or, were they due to my incompetence?

I determined that they weren't moral shortcomings. That lifted a huge burden! Yes, there were challenging circumstances associated with raising four children as a single parent. I may have demonstrated sporadic behavior that, in retrospect, may have been maladaptive, nonsensical, or downright dumb. It did not mean it was deleterious or that I was incompetent. Only after merciless introspection, could I begin to write my much needed mental permission slip granting me forgiveness. It sounded like this: *I am responsible for working two jobs outside the home while trying to raise four young children and for giving the least attention to the child who demanded the least attention. But I am NOT responsible for being a neglectful, unloving, or abusive parent.*

Sometimes we need to re-conceive the past in order to forgive ourselves. Revising my negative self-beliefs about my past allowed me to be at peace with it.

In a Nutshell

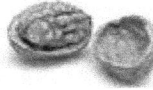

Forgive to live. Let go of grudges for your well-being and longevity.

Forgive others. Adopt the belief that others do not set out to hurt you intentionally and that their behavior is a result of their fear, hurt, pain, or life circumstances. Keep in mind that forgiveness doesn't pardon, condone, or excuse their behavior. It does liberate you from remorse, anger, and vengeance and frees you to continue caring about the other.

Forgive yourself. Humans make mistakes, the vast majority of which are not due to moral ineptitude. People screw up; the Dali Lama, Mother Teresa, Buddha, everybody. Stop beating yourself into a fetal position and learn from it.

Chapter 22: Don't Hesitate— Appreciate!

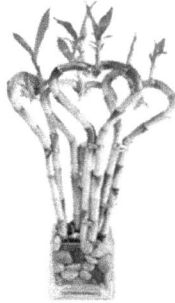

Do you have an attitude of Gratitude?
- SpongeBob SquarePants

Jeanne Calment, a French woman, is my hero. She lived to be 122 and lived independently to the age of 110. Calment was living proof of what longevity experts have concluded: People with good psychological health can slow down the aging process.

"Good psychological health" is described as a positive attitude and the ability to deal with stress. Calment's story prompted me to form this habit:

My Habit: I begin and end each day with gratitude for loved ones, family, friends, and my physical, emotional, intellectual, and financial well-being. I give thanks for living in a country where I am able to earn a good living while helping others and where I am supported and

affirmed by other people. When I focus on those things for which I am grateful, I attract more of them.

Hundreds of studies have documented the social, physical and psychological benefits of gratitude. Some of the top research-based findings that connect gratitude with aging well.

- An interesting study published in the ***American Journal of Cardiology*** reports that gratitude supports cardiovascular and immune system health. People were monitored as they recalled an incident that triggered anger. Then, they were told to reflect on a memory that triggered gratitude. When they did so, their heart, pulse, and respiration rates improved dramatically. When we practice gratefulness, stress is significantly reduced, immune function and overall health is strengthened. Dr. Charles D. Kerns reports that those who are grateful and appreciative live longer.

- In another fascinating longitudinal study, conducted by the University of Kentucky, Catholic nuns who expressed gratitude, happiness, and positive emotions in their earlier years were found to live an average of up to ten years longer than their peers who did not express gratitude.

- HeartMath Institute in California reports that providing a systematic approach to cultivating genuine appreciation reduces stress, chronic disease, nervous system disorders, AND can vastly improve quality of life and promote longevity.

- Studies conducted by Emmons and colleagues at UC Davis suggest that gratitude:

  o Strengthens the immune system, lowers blood pressure, reduces symptoms of illness, and makes you less bothered by aches and pains.

  o Encourages you to exercise more and take better care of your health.

  o Enables you to sleep more soundly.

  o Makes you more resilient.

  o Contributes to an open mind, which improves learning and problem solving.

  o Strengthens relationships. When people express gratitude for each other, they feel closer and more committed.

  o Promotes forgiveness.

  o Causes you to be more helpful, altruistic, and compassionate.

And, gratitude attracts what we want. The book, *The Secret,* explains how the universal law of attraction will bring into your life those things you think about and on which you focus.

If you believe this is so, as I do, wouldn't you want more of those things for which you are thankful?

When you are consciously aware of your blessings and are grateful for them, you are focusing more clearly on what you do want in your life—and are attracting more of those things into your life.

Here is a quick, easy, and re-affirming way to boost your attitude of gratitude:

- Find a quiet space.

- Set a timer for 2 minutes.

- Quickly note **everything** you can think of for which you are grateful, including your unique talents, skills, and accomplishments.

- At the end of 2 minutes, reflect on your list and grant yourself permission to feel good about those things.

If in reviewing your list, it looks short to you, consider this:

> If you have never experienced the horror of war, the solitude of prison, the pain of torture, or were not close to death from starvation, then you have more to be grateful for than 500 million people in the world.

Spend a few minutes at the beginning or at the end of each day, reviewing your list and adding to it based on the previous 24 hours.

In a Nutshell

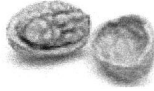

Practicing gratitude has social, physical, psychological and intellectual benefits.

A grateful life is a longer life.

By focusing on those things for which you are grateful, you attract more of them.

Chapter 23: Live on Purpose

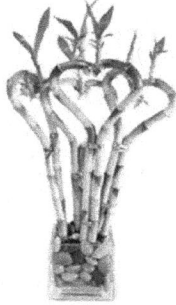

Love is a grave mental disease.
- Plato

Lovelessness is a grave invitation.
- Filomena

Longevity presents a dilemma. The potential for an active, healthy old age is high. So, too, are the terrifying and potentially costly consequences of increased life expectancy. Dementia, Alzheimer's Disease, and a loss of independence are high on the list of concerns of many. These age-related possibilities require constant care and help with the most fundamental activities of daily life. My solution: Live with a purpose of caring for others so that you will not end your life in the care of others. I advocate living on purpose, not just because a noble purpose jump starts your day, but because there is some pretty solid research pointing to the longevity effects of having a purpose.

According to the Dana Foundation, a private philanthropic organization that supports brain research through grants and educates the public about the successes and potential of brain research, mid- and late-life social engagement through volunteering or giving back is associated with better cognitive and physical health and greater longevity.

In fact, loss of identity or feelings of purposelessness or loss of identity due to retirement or physical limitations has been linked to Alzheimer's disease. New research published in the journal, *Archives of General Psychiatry*, assessed more than 900 elderly people whose average age was 80. The researchers found that people who agreed with statements such as, "I feel good when I think of what I have done in the past and what I hope to do in the future" and "I have a sense of direction and purpose in life" were less likely to develop Alzheimer's than those who did not agree.

Loss of purpose or identity can lead to depression. Depression not only makes you feel sick, with aches, pains, and fatigue, it actually makes physical health worse. Depression also gets in the way of memory and concentration. In fact, it can have such an impact on thinking that it's sometimes mistaken for dementia.

So, how can you live a more purposeful life? Just ask and answer the following three questions:

• What is the difference you want to make in the world?

• What do you have going for you that you can tap into to make that difference? What are your unique talents, skills, abilities, or experiences?

• Refer to your gratitude list (chapter 22). How can you use your special skills/experiences/natural abilities to make a positive difference?

There are limitless ways to live on purpose. My next door neighbor volunteers to chauffeur people in our community who are elderly, ill, or facing personal difficulties to their appointments. He is also the first to offer a ride back and forth to the airport whenever anyone is leaving town. His wife volunteers to dog-sit for community pooches and also voluntarily manages homes when the snowbirds move North for the summer. Another neighbor picks up the unsold produce at a local farm market and delivers it to food banks and soup kitchens in the area. I lead an aquatics class on Tuesdays and a weight training/core exercise class on Thursdays. My husband meets with the men at a local assisted living facility twice a week to lead them in activities designed to improve cognition.

What are you good at? How can you pay it back or pay it forward? Some suggestions:

- Be kind to others. Little acts of kindness make a huge difference!

- Just show up! Be there for the people you love. And, be there for people in need, especially when you do not want to be there.

- Be a big brother or a big sister. Or offer a practical workshop at a center for disadvantaged youth: How to interview to get a job, or How to manage on $___/week, or any "how to" that you personally have mastered that might help them.

- Listen up! We all hunger to be heard. Nourish those you encounter with generous listening; it is an act of love.

- Visit the homebound.

- Teach English as a second language.

- Sing in the church choir.

- Promote a cause; breast cancer awareness, feeding the hungry, the March of Dimes, etc. The opportunities are endless.

My Habit: I live to make a difference in the world. I start each day with the intention of doing something that makes another person's life easier, happier, or healthier.

In a Nutshell

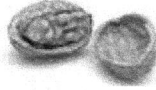

Loss of identity or feelings of purposelessness due to retirement or physical limitations have been linked to Alzheimer's Disease, mental decline and depression.

The antidote is to find a purpose: a way to make a difference in the world.

Pay it forward. Perform daily acts of kindness.

Chapter 24: Think and Act Outside the Box to Stay Outside the Box

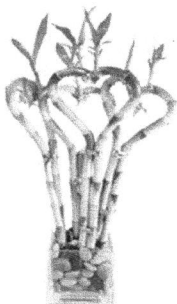

It's not that I'm afraid to die,
I just don't want to be there when it happens.
- Woody Allen

Let me close this segment of the book about living longer with my philosophy about death: I don't believe in dying. I've never spoken to anyone who has done it well. As far as I am concerned death is a rumor created by people who want an excuse to lay down—permanently. I don't intend to do it. Besides, I can't die now. I'm writing this book and it would ruin my reputation for longevity and dramatically limit sales.

Dying is a very depressing, disappointing, and dismal affair. My advice is to avoid it as long as you possibly can by adopting the anti-aging habits offered in this book. Die? That is the last thing I'll do. I want nothing whatsoever to do with it. I suggest that you, too, avoid that box at all costs!

Instead, spend your time thinking and acting outside the box. Do and say things that are outside of societal norms. That way you'll be a source of laughter and ridicule to the living and you will also have lots of time to conjure up inappropriate things to say at their funerals. Comments like what I'm planning to say to my 99-year-old neighbor who is a health nut: *Betcha you felt stupid lying in the hospital dying of nothing!* You too can join me in my quest to put funeral directors out of business.

Here are five ways to think and act differently that are life-enhancing. OK, OK, no one ever did a scientific study to prove these practices lead to greater longevity. However, no dead person ever reported that they hastened their demise. AND, I can attest to the fact that they make life more interesting and enjoyable.

Tell Yourself the Truth—it has the same effect as running naked. Health comes from the root word, to be whole. A profound sense of living authentically can enhance health. We are all unique and by looking inside to connect with your true self you can free yourself to express your fondest hopes and dreams. We need to let go of our long-held feelings of guilt that we feel when we let the world see the truth of who we are without pretense or shame.

One of my truths is this*: Positive attention is a rare, yet inexpensive, high. I am an addict.* Yeah, I run 5 miles every day, lift weights that equal the weight of one of the Olsen twins, and do crunches until I'm so weak I have to signal the attendant at the gym to help me into the sitting position. AND, to tell the truth, I am not entirely driven by the physical/mental fitness benefits. I want to look good and do my best for others. I'm happily married. Whether you are or you aren't, it doesn't matter. We all like lookin' good! It's ok to tell the truth about it. Now that I've fessed up, I feel as if I've just streaked nude across a beautiful poppy-filled field!!!

Avoid Stinkin' Thinkin'. Let's say you eat healthy and occasionally allow yourself a forbidden treat. Then you nag yourself constantly about it. You say things to yourself such as *I should have resisted that,* or *I shouldn't have eaten that.* Or you work out nearly every day, but take two days off every week or so. Then you fret that you'll lose muscle tone telling yourself *I should do double the work tomorrow,* or *I shouldn't be so lazy.* Or, perhaps, you practice meditation for 15 minutes every day, yet you give the universal hand signal and threaten bodily harm to anybody who doesn't drive according to your personal traffic regulations, screaming epithets about the driver's parentage. Then you tell yourself that *I should be more compassionate* or *I shouldn't be so impatient.*

"Shoulding" can destroy the health you build by being physically active by what you do with your mind. When you should on yourself and others you are engaging in stinkin' thinkin': sending crappy messages that negatively influence your thoughts and actions, bias your expectations and influence your behavior. I have a sign in my office, **I won't should on myself today**. Someone who works for me crept in during the night and scrawled on the bottom *"and you won't should all over me either."*

Don't take yourself seriously, no one else does. I spent nearly four decades of my life worrying about what others thought of me. I kicked myself about the head and shoulders for looking bad: making some big mistakes, botched decisions, and regretful alliances. Then, at around 40 years old, I discovered two things: 1) That kind of thinking is narcissistic. Not that I was vain, I was just overly self-absorbed. 2) Even though the voices in my head may not be real, they have some good ideas. One of which is that most of life's major screw ups are perfect fodder for some pretty funny stories where the joke is on you.

My life has been one great big joke.

A dance that's walked,

A song that's spoke,

I laugh so hard I almost choke,

When I think about myself.

Maya Angelou

According to anthropologist, Gil Greengross, who published a study in the ***Journal of Evolutionary Psychology***, self-deprecating humor can be an especially reliable indicator, not only of general intelligence and verbal creativity, but also of moral virtues such as humility. Greengross studied the role of humor in sexual selection for two years and was "surprised" at how often self-deprecating humor was used. Personally, I just love it when I discover a sexual attractor that is smart, quick, and funny. I always thought I was such a good lover because I practiced a lot on my own. I discovered too late that being a hot number has more to do with putting myself down than turning myself on!!!

I could write a whole book filled with hilarious self-deprecation if I could only get around to it. I know my apathy causes me problems, but I don't care.

Get the hell out of your driveway. This practice is based on a study published in the ***American Journal of Geriatric Psychiatry*** that measured mobility: the degree to which people age, based on how they get around in their environment and how much they see beyond their own home. The research revealed that people who never leave their home environment during a week are twice as likely to develop Alzheimer's over a five-year period as those who traveled out of town. People who did not go beyond their driveway or front yard were also more likely to develop mild cognitive impairment. So, take off and discover new horizons while you can still recognize them.

- If you travel the same route for routine shopping trips and visits, consciously choose a different one.

- Find a theater, event, park, lake, stream, or historical site that is nearby that you have never visited. Go!

- If you save $2 a day for three years, you can go anywhere in the world. Most places will take much less than three year's of savings.

- Don't be deterred by fear. There aren't that many dangerous places in the world. True, there are a few war-torn areas or places where citizens are taking to the streets in rebellion. They would not make good vacation spots. But the list of places to avoid is short and the list of incredible places is long.

Do at least one outrageous thing every day. It's best to avoid actions that are illegal or immoral (although the death sentence is a way to permanently halt aging). Just a few of the "out of the box" things I've experimented with:

- Wear a tiara, a Viking hat, a garland of flowers, or other unique head gear. It is liberating, fun, and gives others a lift as well.

- Take a bunch of flowers with you to a mall. Give them to people, one at a time, with a wish for their well-being.

- Break into spontaneous dance. Recently, I was at a rockin' concert at a retirement community and the audience sat placidly listening to some of the best rock and roll I'd heard in ages. These were some of the same people who danced with abandon and dressed in little more than bandaids during the Woodstock era. It must have taken considerable restraint to sit still. Once I got up and started dancing in the aisle, others joined the joy. Dance, dance, dance, like no one is looking!!!

• Write a poem about one of your friends and recite it to him or her.

• Have a slumber party. One of my friends invited six of her friends for a sleep-over the night before the royal wedding of William and Kate. They stayed up all night and were still in their jammies, drinking mimosas and eating crumpets when the wedding started at 4:30 a.m.

• Get a dummy. I studied a book, *Ventriloquism for Dummies*. Then went to e-Bay and bought a puppet, Dr. Payne. I have a blast with Dr. Jayne Payne. She has become an international expert on sex and the older woman. She cracks me up. And, it is a lot more fun than talking to my hand. You can meet Dr. Payne at www.stayoung4ever.org.

One of the great advantages of being an older citizen is that you can get away with so much more than a younger person. The bizarre things you say and do are not only fun for you, they are immensely entertaining for others.

In closing this chapter, I would like to offer just one caveat. Never, never, report that you have seen or made a trip on a flying saucer. If you do, you will be branded a crazy old coot and, worst yet, an uneducated ranch hand from some Southern state.

Section V:
Fantastic Factoids

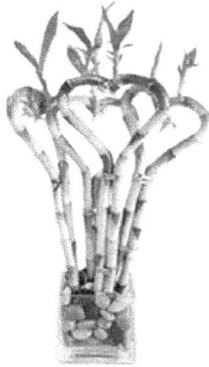

Easy to digest research summaries to sustain your healthy habits and achieve your longevity goals.

Fantastic Factoids

Head Games: How to care for, feed, and train your brain to be smart for life.

Findings: **Sleep can keep you young**. A study has shown that stress increases the energy demands of your stem cells resulting in elevated production of reactive metabolites that can directly damage DNA.

So what? A good night's sleep (45 minutes of sleep for every hour you are awake) aids stem cell ability to efficiently repair DNA damage and increases tissue ability to maintain and repair itself as you age.

Source: German Cancer Research Center (Deutsches Krebsforschungszentrum, DKFZ) as reported in Science Daily Feb 2015.

***

Findings: **Dementia: Walk it off.** New research suggests that walking at least six miles per week may protect brain size and in turn, preserve memory in old age.

So What? Study author Kirk I. Erickson, Ph.D.,University of Pittsburgh, reports that brain size shrinks in late adulthood, which can cause memory problems. Physical exercise in older adults is a promising approach for preventing dementia and Alzheimer's disease.

Source: A study published in the October 13, 2010, online issue of *Neurology®,* the medical *Journal of the American Academy of Neurology.*

***

Findings: **Meditation can keep the aging brain sharp.**

So What? This study was focused on the association between age and gray matter. Scientists compared 50 people who had meditated for years and 50 who did not. Participants in both groups showed a loss of gray matter as they aged. But the researchers report that the decline in the volume of gray matter was not as significant in the meditators.

Source: **Frontiers in Psychology Journal**, Feb 2015 article. Study reported by Dr. Florian Kurth, co-author and postdoctoral fellow at the UCLA Brain Mapping Center as reported in Science Daily.

***

Findings: **Milk may help ward off cognitive decline.**

So What? Researchers found that participants who had indicated they drank milk recently had higher levels of glutathione in their brains. Glutathione helps stave off oxidative stress and the resultant damage caused by reactive chemical compounds produced during the normal metabolic process in the brain. Oxidative stress is associated with a number of different diseases and conditions, including Alzheimer's and Parkinson's diseases.

Source: University of Kansas Medical Center. "Milk could be good for your brain." As reported in Science Daily, March 2015.

***

Findings: **Computerized brain fitness training works.**

So What? UCLA researchers found that older adults who regularly engaged in a brain fitness program on a computer demonstrated significantly improved memory and language skills.

Source: Research conducted by Dr. Karen Miller, associate clinical professor, Semel Institute for Neuroscience and Human Behavior at UCLA and Dr. Gary Small, professor of Psychiatry and Biobehavioral Sciences at the Semel Institute, presented Aug. 2012 at the annual convention of the American Psychological Association, as reported online in Science Daily.

***

Findings: **Regular aerobic exercise can keep your brain sharp.**

So what? According to a study published inthe ***British Journal of Sports Medicine***, regular aerobic exercise seems to boost the size of the area of the brain involved in verbal memory and learning among women whose intellectual capacity has been affected by age. The researchers recommend regular aerobic exercise to stave off mild cognitive decline and overall brain health

Source: Science Daily, April 2014.

Fantastic Factoids

Food for Life: How to fill your tank with high octane fuel that fires up your engine, fights obesity and fends off disease.

Findings: **Two studies to frighten you out of your "happy hour"**

> 1.   Findings: **Drinking just one or two alcoholic drinks a day linked to liver disease**. According to the World Health Organization, excessive alcohol drinking is the most common cause of cirrhosis worldwide.
>
> Source: European Association for the Study of the Liver April 25,   2015
>
> 2.   Findings: **Health benefits of even light drinking may be limited to women 65 and over** and even then may have been exaggerated. According to the **British Medical Journal**, the protective effects of light drinking may be exaggerated by "selection biases" in studies that could skew results. For instance, including former (potentially heavy) drinkers in non-drinking groups or not taking full account of other unmeasured (confounding) factors.

Source: **British Medical Journal**, February 10, 2015.

So what? High alcohol consumption has been associated with more than 200 acute and chronic conditions. Globally, more than three million deaths each year are attributed to alcohol. There is also concern about increasing alcohol consumption among older people and the risk of alcohol-related problems due to impaired metabolism of alcohol with age.

***

Findings: **High Fructose Corn Syrup Raises Risk of Cardiovascular Disease.** A study from the University California Davis has shown for the first time that there is a "dose-dependent" relationship between the amount of the sugar consumed, and the increasing risk of cardiovascular disease. The study's participants were given drinks sweetened with low, medium and high amounts of high-fructose corn syrup. The greater the intake of the sugar, the greater the increase in the measured risk factors for cardiovascular disease.

So what? The study's lead researcher Kimber Stanhope says, "These findings clearly indicate that humans are acutely sensitive to the harmful effects of excess dietary sugar over a broad range of consumption levels."

Source: Henry Sobo, M.D., optimalhealth@optonline.net Medical Director, Integrative, Alternative, Anti-Aging Medicine.

***

Findings: **Two studies reveal: Eat better, live longer.**

    1. Findings: **Diets high in fruit, vegetables, whole grains and nuts one of several factors to lower first-time stroke risk.** Eating Mediterranean or DASH-style diets, regularly engaging in physical activity and keeping your blood pressure under control can lower your risk of a first-time stroke.

    So what? James Meschia, M.D., lead author of the study and professor and chairman of neurology at the Mayo Clinic in Jacksonville, Florida says; "We have a huge opportunity to improve how we prevent new strokes, because the risk factors that can be changed or controlled, especially high blood pressure, which account for 90 percent of strokes." The updated guidelines recommend these tips to lower risk:

- Eat a Mediterranean or DASH-style diet, supplemented with nuts.

- Don't smoke.

- Monitor high blood pressure at home with a cuff device.

- Manage your weight.

- Reduce the amount of sodium in your diet.

- Visit your healthcare provider annually for blood pressure evaluation.

Source: American Heart Association, October 29, 2014

2. Findings: **Eating a Mediterranean diet is associated with longer telomeres.** Telomeres sit on the end of chromosomes (like the plastic tips on the end of shoelaces), stopping them from fraying and scrambling the genetic codes they contain. Telomeres shorten progressively throughout life and gradually shorten life. The Mediterranean diet consists of a high intake of vegetables, fruits, nuts, legumes (such as peas, beans and lentils), unrefined grains, olive oil, a low intake of saturated fats, a moderately high intake of fish, a low intake of dairy products, meat and poultry, and regular but moderate intake of alcohol (specifically wine with meals).

So what? A study led by Immaculata De Vivo, Associate Professor at Brigham and Women's Hospital and Harvard Medical School showed that greater adherence to the Mediterranean diet was significantly associated with longer telomeres. De Vivo reports, "our results further support the benefits of adherence to the Mediterranean diet for promoting health and longevity."

Source: *British Medical Journal*, December 3, 2014.

***

Findings: **Three easy secrets to healthy eating.** A new study analyzed 112 studies that collected information about healthy eating behaviors and found that most healthy eaters did so because a restaurant, grocery store, school cafeteria, or spouse made foods like fruits and vegetables visible and easy to reach (convenient), enticingly displayed (attractive), and appear like an obvious choice (normal).

So what? Think of the kitchen fruit bowl. A fruit bowl makes fruit more convenient, attractive, and normal to eat than if the same fruit were in the bottom of the refrigerator. Better still, don't bring unhealthy foods into your home at all. It makes them **less** visible/convenient, attractive, and normal.

Source: Cornell Food & Brand Lab, April 29, 2015.

***

Findings: **These seven foods can curb your appetite and keep you feeling full longer:**

- **Protein:** Add one protein to breakfast to improve satiety and diet quality.

- **Whole Grains and Fiber:** Oats increase appetite-control hormones up to four hours after a meal.

- **Eggs:** Eating one egg with breakfast will help to reduce hunger between meal times.

- **Almonds:** The healthy fats in almonds decrease hunger and improve dietary vitamin E intake.

- **Pulses:** Pulses include dried peas, edible beans, lentils, and chickpeas. They are very high in protein and low in fat, and are proven to contribute to a feeling of fullness.

- **Saffron Extract:** This extract is shown to have a beneficial effect on appetite, mood, and behaviors relating to snacking

- **Korean Pine Nut Oil:** This nut has high levels of healthy all-natural fats, which are shown to release the satiety hormone cholecystokinin.

So what? Not feeling full after or between meals can result in overeating. Studies that show eating the seven foods listed above may help curb appetite and keep one feeling fuller longer.

Source: *Food Technology Magazine*, October 2014, published by the Institute of Food Technologists (IFT).

***

Findings: **The dark side of chocolate is healthy**. A research team including Prof. Diederik Esser of the Top Institute Food and Nutrition and the Division of Human Nutrition at Wageningen University, both in the Netherlands, has discovered why dark chocolate is good for you. It may reduce the risk of atherosclerosis, the thickening and hardening of the arteries, by restoring flexibility of the arteries and preventing white blood cells from sticking to the blood vessel walls.

So what? In addition to lowering your risk of atherosclerosis, a condition that can be caused by arterial stiffness and white blood cell adhesion, other research has linked chocolate consumption to many other health benefits. Last year, a study suggested that drinking two cups of hot chocolate a day may prevent memory decline while a 2012 study found that eating moderate amounts of chocolate could reduce the risk of stroke.

Source: *Medical News Today*, February 28, 2014.

Fantastic Factoids

Kick Start Your Heart: How to tap into the life-long and long-life benefits of exercise.

Findings: **The heart is forgiving—you can undo heart disease risk by changing lifestyle.** When adults in their 30s and 40s decide to drop unhealthy habits that are harmful to their heart and embrace healthy lifestyle changes, they can control and potentially even reverse the natural progression of coronary artery disease. In a study published June 30, 2014 in the journal *Circulation*, Bonnie Spring, lead investigator of the study and a professor of preventive medicine at Northwestern University Feinberg School of Medicine, said: "You're not doomed if you've hit young adulthood and acquired some bad habits. You can still make a change and it will have a benefit for your heart."

So what? Scientists examined healthy lifestyle behaviors and coronary artery calcification and artery thickening among the more than 5,000 people. The healthy lifestyle factors assessed were: not being overweight/obese, being a non-smoker, being physically active, having low alcohol intake, and a healthy diet. Each increase in healthy lifestyle factors was associated with reduced odds of detectable coronary artery calcification and lower intima-media thickness, two key markers of cardiovascular disease that can predict future cardiovascular events.

"This finding is important because it helps to debunk two myths held by some health care professionals," Spring said. "The first is that it's nearly impossible to change patients' behaviors. Yet, we found that 25 percent of adults made healthy lifestyle changes on their own. The second myth is that the damage has already been done—adulthood is too late for healthy lifestyle changes to reduce the risk of developing coronary artery disease. Clearly**, that's incorrect. Adulthood is not too late for healthy behavior changes to help the heart."**

The bad news: Scientists also found that if people drop healthy habits or pick up more bad habits as they age, there is measurable, detrimental impact on their coronary arteries. If you don't keep up a healthy lifestyle, you'll see the evidence in terms of your risk of heart disease.

Source: Northwestern University, June 30, 2014.

***

Findings: **Healthy lifestyle choices may dramatically reduce risk of heart attack in men.** Following a healthy lifestyle, including maintaining a healthy weight and diet, exercise, not smoking and moderating alcohol intake, could prevent four out of five coronary events in men, according to a new study.

So what? Researchers examined a population of 20,721 healthy Swedish men aged 45-79 years of age and followed them for 11 years. Men in the study with the lowest risk were non-smokers, who walked or cycled for at least 40 minutes per day, exercised at least one hour per week, had a waist circumference below 37.4 inches. They consumed moderate amounts of alcohol, and followed a healthy diet with a regular consumption of fruits, vegetables, legumes, nuts, reduced-fat dairy products, whole grains, and fish. The researchers found a clear reduction in risk for heart attack for each individual lifestyle factor the participants practiced.

Source: American College of Cardiology, September 22, 2014.

***

<u>Findings</u>: **People with Type 2 Diabetes Should Exercise After Dinner.** Individuals with type 2 diabetes have heightened amounts of sugars and fats in their blood, which increases their risks for cardiovascular diseases such as strokes and heart attacks.

<u>So what?</u> Exercise is a popular prescription for individuals suffering from the symptoms of Type 2 diabetes, but little research has explored whether these individuals receive more benefits from working out before or after dinner. Now, researchers at the University of Missouri have found that individuals with Type 2 diabetes can lower their risks of cardiovascular diseases more effectively by exercising after a meal. Participants who exercised 45 minutes after eating dinner, performing resistance exercises such as leg curls, seated calf raises and abdominal crunches were able to reduce both sugar and fat levels.

<u>Source</u>: University of Missouri-Columbia, February 18, 2015.

***

<u>Findings</u>: **Sitting is the new smoking**. Studies have shown that sitting for extended periods of time every day can increase the risk of several health issues, such as heart disease, diabetes and premature death. The study used data from more than 3,200 people who participated in the U.S. National Health and Nutrition Examination Survey. The study found that standing more may not be enough to offset the dangers of sitting for too long; but short bursts of light activities, such as walking, cleaning, and gardening can boost the longevity of people who are sedentary for more than half of their day.

<u>So what?</u> Trading two minutes of sitting for two minutes of light-intensity activity each hour lowered the risk of premature death by 33 percent, the study revealed.

Source: University of Utah School of Medicine, news release, April 30, 2015 as reported by MedLinePlus HealthDay.

***

Findings: **Regular aerobic exercise boosts memory area of brain in older women.** A study published online in the *British Journal of Sports Medicine*, reports that regular aerobic exercise seems to boost the size of the area of the brain involved in verbal memory and learning among women whose intellectual capacity has been affected by age.

So what? Aerobic exercise seems to be able to slow the shrinkage and maintain the volume of the hippocampus in a group of women who are at risk of developing dementia. Researchers recommend regular aerobic exercise to stave off mild cognitive decline, which is especially important, given the mounting evidence showing that regular exercise is good for cognitive function and overall brain health and the rising toll of dementia. The number of those afflicted is set to rise to more than 115 million by 2050.

Source: *British Medical Journal*, April 8, 2014 as reported by U.S. National Library of Medicine, National Institutes of Health.

***

Findings: **Centers for Disease Control reports U.S. Life Expectancy Hits Record High of Nearly 79 Years.**

So what? The increased life expectancy is likely due to Americans living healthier lifestyles. Nuff said!!!!

Source: HealthDay, Wednesday, October 8, 2014.

***

Findings: **To reap the brain benefits of physical activity, just get moving.** Everyone knows that exercise makes you feel more mentally alert at any age. But do you need to follow a specific training program to improve your cognitive function? Science has shown that the important thing is just to get moving. It's that simple.

So what? A study conducted at the Institut universitaire de gériatrie de Montréal (IUGM), an institution affiliated with Université de Montréal, by Dr. Nicolas Berryman, PhD, Exercise Physiologist, under the supervision of Dr. Louis Bherer, PhD, and Dr. Laurent Bosquet, PhD, studied the impact of exercise on the brain's executive functions. The executive functions allow us to continue reacting effectively to a changing environment. We use them to plan, organize, develop strategies, pay attention to and remember details, and manage time and space. For a long time, it was believed that only aerobic exercise could improve executive functions. More recently, science has shown that strength training also leads to positive results. These new findings suggest that structured activities that aim to improve gross motor skills can also expand executive functions, which decline as we age. Remember you have the power to improve your physical and cognitive health at any age and you have many avenues to reach this goal.

Source: Université de Montréal   October 29, 2014, Study published in the *Journal American Aging Association.*

Fantastic Factoids

The Joy Factor: How to capture the joy of a love affair with life.

Findings: **Having a sense of meaning and purpose in your life might do more than you think.**

So what? Having a purpose might do more than just give you focus, it might help you live longer, too. A study, involving more than 9,000 British people averaging 65 years of age, found that those who professed to feeling worthwhile and having a sense of purpose in life were less likely to die during the more than eight years the researchers tracked them.

Source: University College London, news release, Nov. 6, 2014; Eric Kim, Ph.D. candidate, psychology, University of Michigan, Ann Arbor; James Maddux, Ph.D., university professor emeritus, psychology, George Mason University, Fairfax, Va.; Nov. 3, 2014, *Proceedings of the National Academy of Sciences*, online as reported in Med Line.

***

Findings: **Taking in such spine-tingling wonders as the Grand Canyon, Sistine Chapel ceiling, or Schubert's 'Ave Maria' may give a boost to the body's defense mechanisms.**

So what? Researchers have linked positive emotions, especially the awe we feel when touched by the beauty of nature, art, and spirituality, with lower levels of pro-inflammatory cytokines, which are proteins that signal the immune system to work harder. "Our findings demonstrate that positive emotions are associated with the markers of good health," said Jennifer Stellar, a postdoctoral researcher at the

University of Toronto and lead author of the study, which she conducted while at UC Berkeley.

Source: University of California - Berkeley, February 3, 2015 as reported online in Science Daily.

***

Findings: **Love transforms your brain**. When you fall in love with someone, parts of your brain are activated.

So what? People in love have higher levels of dopamine, which is linked to pleasure, desire and euphoria. Studies report that people in positive, healthy relationships live longer, are happier, wiser, and have better mental health. Through MRI scans, researchers have found that when we fall in love, the frontal cortex, the area of the brain that's responsible for judgment, shuts down. So when you are in love, you are less likely to be critical or skeptical of the person you care about. In healthy relationships, holding on to your partner's hand is enough to keep you from stressing, lower your blood pressure, ease your physical pain, and improve your health.

Source: Psych Central, April 28, 2015.

***

Findings: **A happy or sad way of walking actually affects your mood.**

So what? Researchers have shown that when participants walked with a slump-shouldered depressed walking style, itcreated a depressed mood. Those with a happy way of walking reported more positive events. A light walk, shoulders back, lively gait seems like a very inexpensive anti-depressant!

Source: A study published in the *Journal of Behavior Therapy and Experimental Psychiatry* by CIFAR Senior Fellow Nikolaus Troje of Queen's University, as reported online in Science Daily, October 15, 2014.

Findings: **Mindfulness training linked with reduced stress and stress-related disease outcomes.**

So what? When you experience stress, activity in the prefrontal cortex (which is responsible for conscious thinking and planning) decreases while activity in the regions that quickly activate your body's stress response increases. Studies suggest that mindfulness reverses these patterns during stress and can turn down the biological stress response, thus reducing the risk of stress-related diseases such as depression and heart disease.

Source: Carnegie Mellon University as reported online in Science Daily, February 12, 2015.

A Final Word

Here is a final "Fascinating Factoid." The number of American centenarians has been doubling every decade since the 1950s; by 2050, the number of centenarians living in the US is expected to pass one million. Given that you've completed *Anti-Aging Habits*, you are likely to be among them!

Most people do not revel in the thought of living to be 100 or older. For many, aging is synonymous with aches and pains, forgetfulness and loneliness. It is inevitable that you're going to get older. How you age is anything but inevitable.

None of us will get out of this world alive. But we can go out having lived a fit, fulfilling life thanks to anti-aging habits that keep our minds sharp, our bodies fit, our organs functioning properly, and our spirits high.

I just celebrated my 77th birthday. I am the fittest I have ever been and I live every day to its fullest. True, I could run faster when I was younger, but I would never trade that for the muscle strength, flexibility, vivacity, and knowledge I have today. For me, in many ways, life continues to get better as the years go by. I hope you find the same.

Aging seems to be the only available way to live a long life. There are no guarantees relative to the number of years you will live. What **is** certain is this: You won't find the secret to longevity in fad diets, supplements, or expensive spas. Those are marketing ploys that ply you with promise. You have the secret. It's this: the fountain of youth springs from your head.

The premise behind *Anti-Aging Habits* is to die young as late as possible. Adopt the habits recommended in this book to maintain your youthful vim, vigor, and vitality as long as you inhabit this earth.

Here is to your good health, energy, enthusiasm, excitement, and the joy of kickin' ass for at least 100 years!